MW00415893

THE
NOCEBO
EFFECT

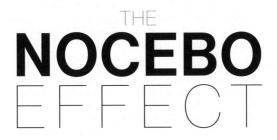

THE
NOCEBO
EFFECT

WHEN WORDS MAKE YOU SICK

Edited by
Michael H. Bernstein, Ph.D.,
Charlotte Blease, Ph.D.,
Cosima Locher, Ph.D., and
Walter A. Brown, M.D.

Mayo Clinic Press

MAYO CLINIC PRESS
200 First St. SW
Rochester, MN 55905
mcpress.mayoclinic.org

The information in this book is true and complete to the best of our knowledge. This book is intended as an informative guide for those wishing to learn more about health issues. It is not intended to replace, countermand or conflict with advice given to you by your own physician. The ultimate decision concerning your care should be made between you and your doctor. Information in this book is offered with no guarantees. The author and publisher disclaim all liability in connection with the use of this book.

The views expressed are the author's personal views, and do not necessarily reflect the policy or position of Mayo Clinic.

To stay informed about Mayo Clinic Press, please subscribe to our free e-newsletter at mcpress.mayoclinic.org or follow us on social media.

For bulk sales to employers, member groups and health-related companies, contact Mayo Clinic at SpecialSalesMayoBooks@mayo.edu.

Proceeds from the sale of every book benefit important medical research and education at Mayo Clinic.

Cover design by Nikolaas Eickelbeck

Library of Congress Cataloguing in Publication Data
Names: Bernstein, Michael (Michael H.), editor. | Blease, Charlotte, editor. | Locher, Cosima, editor. | Brown, Walter A. (Walter Armin), 1941- editor. | Mayo Clinic, issuing body.
Title: The nocebo effect: when words make you sick / [edited by] Michael Bernstein, Charlotte Blease, Cosima Locher, and Walter Brown.
Description: First edition. | Rochester, MN : Mayo Clinic Press, 2024. | Includes bibliographical references and index. |
Identifiers: LCCN 2023016730 (print) | LCCN 2023016731 (ebook) | ISBN 9798887700243 (hardcover) | ISBN 9798887700250 (ebook)
Subjects: MESH: Nocebo Effect | COVID-19 Vaccines | Disinformation | Vaccine Hesitancy | Patient Harm–psychology | Public Opinion | United States
Classification: LCC RA638 (print) | LCC RA638 (ebook) | NLM WB 330 | DDC 615.3/72–dc23/eng/20231101
LC record available at https://lccn.loc.gov/2023016730
LC ebook record available at https://lccn.loc.gov/2023016731

ISBN: 979-8-88770-024-3 hardcover
ISBN: 979-8-88770-025-0 ebook

Printed in China

First edition: 2024

*We hope that patients will suffer less due
to continued insights into the nocebo
effect. This book is dedicated to them.*

TABLE OF CONTENTS

THE
NOCEBO
EFFECT

INTRODUCTION

Michael H. Bernstein, Charlotte Blease,
Cosima Locher, and Walter A. Brown

THE NOCEBO EFFECT IN OUR CONTEMPORARY
PUBLIC HEALTH LANDSCAPE

In March 2020, the world closed its doors. One country after another instituted lockdown orders to help curb the spread of the COVID-19 virus. At the time of this writing, worldwide there have been more than 686 million confirmed coronavirus cases and more than 6.8 million COVID-19 deaths.[1] Pharmaceutical companies worked tirelessly to develop vaccines, which were ultimately created in record time.

A staggering 12.7 billion doses of the COVID vaccine have been administered around the world, with nearly 613 million doses in the United States alone.[2] Undoubtedly, the vaccine has saved countless lives. While we should appreciate these innovations of modern-day medical science, the vaccine has not been universally accepted, and as Kate MacKrill will explore in Chapter 11 of this book, this may be partially attributed to the *nocebo effect.*

A substantial proportion of the population is wary of the vaccine, and 20 percent of Americans have not received any vaccination, according to the *New York Times* COVID tracker. Concern over adverse effects is fueling resistance. And vaccines do have some specific side effects—meaning symptoms that occur as a direct result of the vaccine ingredients.

Side effects of the COVID vaccine are widely discussed in news outlets. A CNN headline read, "Here's Why That Second Coronavirus Shot Can Be Such a Doozy." A CBS News article, titled "Should You Plan a Sick Day in Case of COVID-19 Vaccine Side Effects?" suggests that people plan for one or two days off work after receiving their shot. One Fox News article quotes a CDC expert who said that "people should be prepared to have . . . a low-grade fever." Countless online discussion boards teem with anecdotes of people feeling sick after getting jabbed.

But lost in this discussion of side effects, and ignored by the CDC, vaccine experts, and the media, is the inconvenient fact that a significant portion of these side effects are not actually caused by the vaccine. Instead, they are the result of our negative expectations, the so-called nocebo effect.

Imagine a world in which side effects of the COVID vaccine were given less attention. How many fewer people would take sick days after getting their shot? How many more people would be willing to get their vaccine in the first place? If your intuition is that we would be a healthier society if we talked less about vaccine side effects, then you understand the power of the nocebo effect.

"NOCEBO EFFECT" IS A DIFFICULT TERM TO DEFINE. It stems from the Latin word *nocere*, which translates roughly as "to harm." Some experts view it as a kind of negative placebo effect in which the outcome is undesirable, such as a headache or stomachache, while the placebo effect, such as feeling less pain or depression, is desirable. No surprise, then, that the nocebo effect has been called "the placebo effect's evil twin." In our view, the nocebo effect can be summarized as "the occurrence of a harmful event that stems from consciously or subconsciously expecting it." The core of the nocebo effect is that adverse health effects occur as a result of negative *expectations*. Expectations come up in everyday conversation, like when you tell a friend that you're stuck in traffic but expect to meet them for dinner in twenty minutes. But it's also an important technical term that academics use (sometimes interchangeably with *expectancy*), and it was popularized by Dr. Irving Kirsch at Harvard University. Expectancies can teach us a lot about our behavior and actions. They are critical to our health and well-being. The nocebo effect, then, can be thought of as the scientific term for saying that when you expect to feel sick, you are more likely to feel sick.

You might be thinking, "Well, obviously! I don't need a book to teach me that." We'd bet the experience of getting your blood drawn *felt* a lot worse than stubbing your toe, even though the raw sensation of stubbing your toe caused more pain. But only one of these events invokes an expectation. You might say to yourself before the needle goes in, "I'm about to feel a burning in my right arm. I want it to be done quickly." And that kind of self-talk makes the experience more uncomfortable, unlike stubbing a toe, which happens without warning and therefore without any kind of expectation. You'd never say, "I'm about to stub my toe, and it's really going to hurt."

Again, none of this is news to you, though it might not be an idea you've verbalized before. We hope to show you just how important and pervasive the effect is, on both a personal and societal level.

THE HISTORY OF NOCEBO RESEARCH: WHERE DID IT COME FROM?

In the 1950s, Dr. Henry Beecher, who served as a physician in World War II, published a series of seminal papers on the placebo effect. Beecher documented instances where he gave wounded soldiers saline—that is, salt water—but told them they were receiving a powerful painkiller. Beecher did not engage in this deception out of cruelty; in fact, it was just the opposite. Dr. Beecher was an anesthesiologist and faced the difficult task of rationing an all-too-limited supply of morphine. What Beecher noticed on the battlefield has sparked seventy years of modern-day science on the placebo effect: soldiers experienced substantial pain relief from the saline.

The field started as just a few papers on the placebo effect, but it has since blossomed into a full-fledged body of theoretical and empirical work. In 2023, scholars gathered for the fourth Society of Interdisciplinary Placebo Studies conference, founded by Dr. Charlotte Blease (a co-editor of this book) and colleagues, and devoted to the study of placebo science. Placebo research has been published in top academic journals, but it has also captured the public imagination, with leading popular press articles in nearly all major media outlets.

The topic of nocebo has emerged largely from work on the placebo effect. And while thorough reviews of nocebo are lacking, it is still a critical factor to consider in patient care. So where did the idea of the nocebo effect originate? The answer is more confusing than you might imagine. We can trace the origin of it back to at least the 1700s.

Franz Mesmer was an eighteenth-century German physician who developed an interesting cure for a range of maladies. Mesmer believed that illnesses could be alleviated by using magnets to govern the flow of fluid in people's bodies. This might seem preposterous, but bear in mind that Mesmer lacked any of our modern-day tools of science and medicine. He lived in an era when leeches, used for bloodletting, were considered therapeutic. Nonetheless, Louis XVI, king of France at the time, was skeptical of Mesmer's claims. He established a commission to investigate, led by Benjamin Franklin. Franklin and the others did what we would now refer to as placebo-controlled studies to, as the commission put it, "separate the effects of the imagination from those attributed to magnetism." The commissioners led patients to believe they were being magnetized even though they weren't. But all the usual magnetism side effects were still present. On one occasion, the commission noted that after a minute a patient began "shivering, [convulsing], with chattering of her teeth, twisting of her arms and trembling of the whole body."[3] It's no surprise, then, that they ultimately concluded that results attributed to Mesmer's treatment were due only to "imagination."

There are two important points to be taken from this story. The first is that Franklin and the other commissioners identified nocebo effects. The side effects experienced by Mesmer's patients were due to the *expectation* of having side effects. Magnetism itself did not cause them, because the patients weren't actually magnetized. The other thing to note here is that treatment effects and side effects go hand in hand. The patient's shivers and convulsions were side effects of a treatment intended to alleviate suffering. They were viewed as integral, but not as therapeutic in themselves. That is important to consider as you read this book. Nocebo effects are often about side effects, and divorcing the good and bad from treatment is not so easy. If it were, you wouldn't worry so much about that pill causing fatigue, weight gain, or irritability.

Fast-forward about 150 years, to the mid-1900s. One of the top medical journals in the United States, the *Journal of the American Medical Association*, published some papers that documented the existence of side effects among patients who received a placebo. Dr. Harold Diehl, a physician who focused on treating the common cold, seems to have been the first to observe that certain people fall ill after taking a placebo. He conducted double-blind vaccine trials to test treatments for the common cold and noticed a small portion of people had negative reactions to a lactose pill[4] or a placebo vaccine.[5] Though these findings were reported in his paper, little attention was paid to them. In the 1950s, Stewart Wolf, a pioneer in studying the placebo effect, reported on an experiment in which hospital inpatients with anxiety were given a real drug or a placebo to help quell their nervousness.[6] In Wolf's paper, we see for the first time a more thorough discussion of negative placebo reactions. Wolf and his co-author, Ruth Pinsky, wrote: "Minor reactions—nausea, drowsiness, lightheadedness, and palp[it]ation—were often noticed on placebo administration." They reported that one patient even developed "a diffuse itchy [rash after] 10 days of taking pills. . . . The patient firmly refused to try another batch of pills. Later it was learned that the rash had developed while she was taking placebos."

Yet another patient had severe gastric pain and diarrhea after taking the placebo.

At this point, the story of nocebo returns to World War II anesthesiologist Henry Beecher. In a landmark paper that played a major role in paving the way forward for placebo research, Beecher devoted a section to what he called the "toxic" effects of a placebo. In Beecher's words, "Not only do placebos produce beneficial results, but . . . they have associated toxic effects."[7] According to Beecher, there were thirty-five different side effects caused by placebos, such as dry mouth, nausea, and headache.

You might think that it was Beecher, or perhaps Diehl or Wolf, who coined the term "nocebo" to label their observations. However, it was actually Walter Kennedy, who first used the word "nocebo" in 1961, nearly thirty years after Diehl's first paper. Even at that point, formal research into nocebo languished. According to a database of placebo and nocebo research kept by the Society of Interdisciplinary Placebo Studies, only two articles on nocebo were published in the twenty-five years after Kennedy's paper. However, parallel to the spike in placebo research over the past couple of decades, nocebo research has also proliferated. Recently, studies have documented the critical role of nocebos in treatment side effects, explored the psychological and social processes that produce nocebo effects, and suggested how they can be minimized.

PSYCHOGENIC ILLNESSES: FROM THE JUNE BUG TO HAVANA SYNDROME

The mind's unfortunate ability to cause suffering is well established, and this phenomenon lies at the heart of the nocebo effect. One such example, known as "The June Bug," occurred in a textile factory in the United States in the early 1960s. Many employees began to feel dizzy and had an upset stomach. Some people vomited. Rumors of a mysterious bug that was biting employees began to circulate, and eventually sixty-two people who worked at the factory became ill. So what were these mysterious bugs? According to experts, they were nothing—literally. The CDC investigated this outbreak, but no bugs or any other cause of the illnesses could be identified. It instead appears to have been a case of what has often been labeled "mass hysteria," though it is now called *psychogenic illness*.

Over the course of history, there have been countless examples of psychogenic illness—sickness caused by belief. Symptoms can range from hysterical laughter to vomiting to seizures. No organic reason for such outbreaks has yet been identified, despite the best attempts of doctors and health professionals. Psychogenic outbreaks trace back as far as the Middle Ages. Aldous Huxley, author of the widely read dystopian novel *Brave New World*, described one such example from the seventeenth century in a lesser-known work titled *The Devils of Loudun*. As Huxley documents, Loudun, France, was home to a serious psychogenic outbreak among nuns, perceived at the time to be caused by demonic possession, symptoms of which included laughing fits and convulsions. It can be considered an early example of the nocebo effect.

But would such a mass outbreak occur today? It might be easier to imagine people from the Middle Ages, or even a half century ago, experiencing this type of bizarre illness than it would be to think of such a thing happening in the twenty-first century. During 2016 and 2017, however, twenty-one American diplomats in Cuba experienced a range of bizarre neurological symptoms such as hearing loss and nausea.[8] News of what came to be known as "Havana Syndrome" spread, and eventually more than two hundred U.S. government personnel in diplomatic missions in several countries became ill.[9] This case was more troubling than just a few individuals who got sick with unexplained symptoms. Speculation quickly mounted regarding nefarious acts by our foes abroad. One leading theory was that the Russian government was releasing invisible microwaves that caused people to get sick. This might sound like a fringe conspiracy theory, but it has been discussed in leading news sources ranging from the *Washington Post* to NPR. In a 2021 meeting, the cause of Havana Syndrome was discussed among the secretary of state, the attorney general, the CIA director, and the FBI director. Would so many high-ranking U.S. officials meet if they believed that Russian interference was off the table as a potential cause?

To be clear, we do not yet know for certain the cause of these neurological conditions. It is even conceivable that the speculation about Russian interference will ultimately prove correct. However, there are plenty of similarities between what happened relatively recently in Cuba and what happened in the past in Loudun, France, and elsewhere. It should be concerning to scientists and the public alike that the *possibility* of a psychogenic reaction is not being taken seriously. As discussed by *New York Times* reporter Serge Schmemann,[10] the person who was hired to oversee the investigation into Havana Syndrome was pushed out of this role because she refused to take psychogenic illness off the menu of potential causes.

Germs are not the only way that illnesses can spread. Psychological outbreaks are very real, and Havana Syndrome fits the same pattern that has been observed so often before. As Mark Twain is alleged to have said, "History does not repeat itself, but it rhymes." Imagine if speculation about Russian interference gained more of a foothold. What if then-president Donald Trump had released inflammatory tweets about it? How would Vladimir Putin have responded? Could this have turned into a global incident? The nocebo effect is powerful indeed.

THE NOCEBO EFFECT AND THE
COST OF MEDICAL CARE

The United States spends $4.3 trillion on healthcare costs annually,[11] which amounts to more than $12,000 per person and nearly 20 percent of GDP. That amount is expected to continue rising through the 2020s. Healthcare spending is substantially higher in the United States compared to other Western countries.[12] And if it seems like the price of your doctor's visit is higher today than in the past, you are not mistaken. From 2000 to 2022, the cost of healthcare services increased by an average of 3.5 percent annually.[13] In other words, you would have to spend $213 today to cover the healthcare services that you would have received for $100 in 2000. This has considerably outpaced the rate of general inflation.

Despite the high cost, healthcare provides many products and services that we, as a country, cherish. Did you fall off a ladder and now can't move your arm? You can simply drive to an emergency department to get an x-ray and bandages. Or if you can't drive, an ambulance will take you. Have you recently been diagnosed with

HIV or hepatitis? You can see a doctor at an infectious disease clinic to discuss medication, lifestyle modifications, and how to protect your loved ones from contracting the illness as well. But, as we all know, medicine is far from perfect. Even aside from systemic concerns like the reimbursement process from insurance companies and overworked providers, the practice of medicine itself can sometimes directly harm patients. Martin Makary and Michael Daniel have argued that medical errors are the third-leading cause of death in the United States.[14] And side effects from medication—something of particular relevance to the topic of this book—are very costly. Between physician visits, going to the hospital, and other such events, drug-related morbidity and mortality cost the United States over $500 billion in 2016.[15] One such cause is labeled "adverse drug reactions" (ADR), which is a fancy way of saying drug side effects. A study from England found that over a six-year period, more than half a million people were admitted to a hospital with an ADR. This means that for every thousand people who went to the hospital, fifteen were there because of an ADR.[16] But were they sick only from the chemical ingredient of the drug, or was their illness due in part to the nocebo effect?

In another study, Widya Insani and colleagues conducted a meta-analysis of ADR studies.[17] A meta-analysis is a big report that synthesizes the results of prior, smaller studies. In this meta-analysis, the authors looked at thirty-three earlier studies of the frequency of ADRs in primary care. About half of the studies were based in Europe, with the other half in the United States and Australia. In total, the rate of ADRs varied widely—from less than 1 percent to 65 percent. This is precisely why a meta-analysis can be so valuable, since any one study is liable to over- or underestimate the true rate. On average, across all the thirty-three trials, Insani and colleagues found a prevalence rate of 8.3 percent. For every hundred patients in primary care, eight experience an adverse drug reaction. While this may seem like a small proportion, in the United States alone there are typically more than 400 million primary care visits per year;[18] 8 percent translates to 32 million ADRs. So it is far from a trivial issue. As Sir William Osler, the father of modern medicine, is credited as saying, "The person who takes medicine must recover twice, once from the disease, and once from the medicine." And a substantial portion of patients who need to recover from the medicine, to use Osler's words, may in fact be recovering from the nocebo effect.

WHY WE ASSEMBLED THIS BOOK

The placebo effect has clearly captured the public imagination, but the equally important nocebo effect has not yet been given its due. That is what we hope to fix here. Aside from a small group of academic psychologists, psychiatrists, and philosophers, few in the health professions are aware of this phenomenon. We think it is virtually unknown to the public.

With this in mind, we asked experts, most known personally to one or more of us, to write about a particular aspect of the nocebo effect. Their contributions cover most of what is known to date about the topic: what the nocebo effect looks like, the mischief it causes, and how it can be managed. After reading their chapters, we hope you agree that understanding what the nocebo effect is, and its implications, is important to us all.

The book is divided into four parts. Part One is devoted to showing how the nocebo effect can impact your health and well-being. We start in Chapter 1 with a discussion of clinical research. For instance, the authors will show that people can experience side effects from taking a placebo and that withdrawing treatment is more painful when a patient knows that treatment is being taken away. Chapter 2 provides a discussion of how the nocebo effect applies to psychotherapy. A therapist's job is to talk to her patient; if words can make you sick, then even a slight faux pas from a therapist can spell bad news for the patient. Chapter 3 returns to the opening of this book by discussing how the nocebo effect interacts with the COVID-19 pandemic.

Part Two takes a deeper dive into why the nocebo effect occurs. Chapter 4 asks, "What is the nocebo effect, exactly?" The author offers a philosophical answer to this question in much more detail than the back-of-the-envelope definition given on page 3. In Chapter 5, we turn to how the nocebo effect works biologically. Chapter 6 looks at two ways the nocebo effect happens psychologically: by amplifying your day-to-day bodily signals and by misattributing them.

Part Three is intended to provide practical advice to patients and providers. It starts, in Chapter 7, by laying out ethical dilemmas that we face when thinking about nocebos. At the core of these ethical challenges is the tension between two difficult-to-reconcile values: that patients should know about the side effects of their treatment, and that patient harm should be minimized. If you get to this point in the book wondering what can be done about the nocebo effect, the following two chapters will be of particular value.

Chapter 8 offers advice to clinicians on how they interact with patients. Chapter 9 can help empower patients to reduce the sting of the nocebo effect when they interact with providers. Nocebo research is in its infancy, so there is little empirical work tackling this topic directly. However, the authors have called on their clinical experience to arm readers with tools for their next doctor's visit.

We end the book in Part Four by zooming out and thinking about the nocebo effect in society at large. Chapter 10 takes a public health perspective. Drawing on research related to high-voltage power lines, it shows that the nocebo effect can occur in response to environmental features. And if you've ever been taken aback by all the side effects listed at the end of a drug commercial, then Chapter 11 will be for you. It presents compelling research showing how the media might be unwittingly causing nocebo effects. The final chapter takes us on a tour of cave-guarding demons, shrinking penises, and sick U.S. intelligence operators to show how the nocebo effect works across cultures.

PART ONE

THE NOCEBO EFFECT
AND YOUR HEALTH

CHAPTER 1

THE NOCEBO EFFECT IN THE CLINIC

Stefanie H. Meeuwis and Andrea W. M. Evers

"First, do no harm" is one of the oldest ethical oaths in the Western world, and doctors have sworn to it for centuries. It is drilled into all medical doctors during their training. Intentional malpractice, the harming of patients, and other forms of wrongdoing can all result in doctors losing their license. But what if clinicians harm their patients unintentionally? There is a form of harm that can cause serious side effects, undermine treatment effects, and result in patients needing more treatment. Yet medical doctors, patients, and even billion-dollar pharmaceutical companies remain mostly unaware of this harm. As you guessed, we are talking about the nocebo effect. The nocebo effect can arise from a doctor's suggestive words or actions, or the patient's own negative expectancies. These expectancies can be about whether a treatment works for a medical condition, but they can also concern side effects.

WHAT HAPPENS WHEN YOU KNOW ABOUT SIDE EFFECTS?

To study the nocebo side effect, Dr. Ajay Gupta and his research team at Imperial College London followed a group of patients who were participating in a large research trial on the efficacy of a statin called atorvastatin.[1] Statins are medicines that lower the cholesterol level in the blood and can prevent the development of cardiovascular diseases such as stroke. But statins have side effects, including muscle pain, cramping, and muscle weakness. To investigate the extent to which these side effects may be nocebo effects, Gupta looked at patients at risk of developing cardiac disease in two phases. In the first phase, patients (and, for that matter, their doctors) were unsure who was receiving the statins and who was receiving the placebo pills. In the second phase, patients did know that they were taking statins. The number of complaints of muscle symptoms that they reported increased by 30 percent. This was just from the knowledge they were taking statins.

Of course, you could reason that the increase in side effects reporting has nothing to do with nocebo effects; it may just be that people feel more certain about why they experience muscle symptoms and feel more at ease reporting them. Perhaps so—but the evidence provided by other research suggests something different. For example, in another study, this time on the topic of sexual functioning,[2] Italian researcher Dr. Nicola Mondaini and his colleagues studied men who suffered from prostate gland enlargement, dividing them into groups and giving each group different information about a drug called finasteride. Doctors commonly prescribe finasteride to treat prostate gland enlargement, but in some cases it can reduce sexual functioning and libido. Mondaini told one of the groups in the study that they might experience side effects that affected sexual functioning; another group was told only that they would get the medicine but not what the side effects were. The researchers then followed everyone over one year to track the number of side effects the study recruits experienced. As the researchers suspected, those who received information about the specific side effects were more likely to suffer from sexual dysfunction and decreased libido. Again, the only difference between groups was *what they were told*, not the drug itself.

Knowing that nocebo effects occur is one thing, but you may ask yourself whether we should care. After all, if medicine helps treat a disease, then surely people will not mind a few more side effects, right? As it turns out, this is not quite true. Side effects are among the primary reasons for quitting a treatment. In the case of statins, the numbers of those who discontinue treatment are especially high. Dr. Peter Penson and his colleagues combined the evidence of many studies to show that up to 78 percent of the people who stopped taking statins discontinued the drug because of adverse effects.[3] Many of the patients were experiencing nocebo effects, though, which essentially means that *they quit because of their negative expectations, not because of the drug.* And quitting a drug is not always a harm-free decision. Stopping treatment can be dangerous: high cholesterol levels in the blood can lead to a heart attack when patients do not take statins to keep their cholesterol level under control. When this is taken into account, the consequences of experiencing nocebo effects can easily turn into a serious matter.

ANTICIPATORY NAUSEA AND LEARNING

If someone experienced side effects in the past, they may be more vulnerable to nocebo effects in the future. People learn to make associations between events, and between feelings and those events. When a person encounters something that reminds them of one of those events, they may reexperience the same feelings they had before as a learned response. For instance, a song that was played at your wedding can make you feel happy for years into the future. But if the song was played at your dad's funeral, you may have the opposite reaction. This can also happen with physical responses and symptoms, as is the case for food and nausea.

The idea that learning can lead to side effects may at first seem outlandish. But just as Pavlov's dogs automatically started to drool in response to the sound of a bell preceding the arrival of food, your physiological response system can actively prepare itself for food digestion.[4] When someone sees, hears, or smells something that they associate with food (such as seeing or hearing a fridge door open, or smelling freshly baked bread), the anticipatory response is triggered and hormones such as insulin are released. That is why you may start salivating when taking a pie out of the oven, even though your body does not yet "need" the saliva for digestion. There is an evolutionary reason for this. When the body is prepared for food intake, it can get the most energy out of the food consumed. In times when food is scarce, this may give an individual better odds of surviving. Similarly, it could be beneficial if physiological response systems that remove harmful substances from the body become active before the harmful substance enters the body. In 2000, Dr. Sibylle Klosterhalfen and her colleagues conducted an experiment at Heinrich Heine University in Düsseldorf, Germany, to demonstrate that anticipatory symptoms are learned responses.[5] They asked participants to sit on a chair that had been placed inside a striped tube that rotated around the participant. The rotation of the tube tricks a person's brain into thinking they are moving when they are not, which can then cause motion sickness. Half the participants in the study drank juice right before sitting in the rotating tube; the other half drank it an hour earlier. Those who drank the juice immediately before rotation developed a clear aversion to its taste: when they were asked to drink the juice again, they consumed less of it than they did before, and less than the participants who had drunk it at an earlier time. This is likely because they associated it with becoming nauseated.

Bad experiences with treatment can lead to associations between nausea and the environment, too. This happens often in treatment of childhood rheumatism. Children with this disease have to take tablets or receive injections of methotrexate (MTX) regularly. Dr. Alex van der Meer and co-workers at University Medical Center Utrecht in the Netherlands looked at the side effects of MTX.[6] They showed that close to one in every three children developed anticipatory nausea. Interestingly, the moment the children experienced nausea varied, but in all instances, they felt nauseated when seeing something that reminded them of getting the drug. Some children became nauseous when they entered the doctor's office, and some when they saw the syringe or tablet. In other cases, the children felt nauseated upon seeing anything yellow, which as you may guess is the color of MTX. Adults may be able to reason they need to suffer through nausea to get better, but this is more difficult to explain to children, especially when they are young. The experience of nocebo side effects could contribute to a general negative attitude toward medicine. This attitude, unfortunately, leaves people even more vulnerable to nocebo effects. Moreover, nocebo effects can go beyond side effects to impact the treatment itself.

BEYOND SIDE EFFECTS

In 2003, Dr. Fabrizio Benedetti and his colleagues at the University of Turin in Italy tested how the context of care contributes to the effects of medicine.[7] To do this, they designed a study in which they compared the effects of treatment information with the effects of medical treatment alone. All patients were in the hospital and received morphine intravenously to manage their pain following an operation. In one group, a doctor came in to tell patients that they would stop the administration of morphine (the researchers called this the "open interruption" group). In the other group, providers stopped morphine administration without telling the patient anything ("hidden interruption"). The results painted a clear picture. The patients who were led to develop negative expectancies—thinking, for example, "The morphine is stopped *now*, therefore my pain will increase"—were in more pain than those who were cut off from morphine without knowing it. That's not all. Patients in the study could request more painkillers if they needed them—and here the contrast between the two groups was even more striking. After the doctor told patients that their morphine would be stopped, fourteen out of sixteen patients requested additional painkillers. In the hidden interruption group, this number was more than halved (only six out of sixteen patients requested painkillers). Not only did the patients who knew the doctor had stopped treatment feel more pain but they also needed more drugs to cope with it.

What Benedetti's study demonstrates is that negative expectancies can hamper pain relief. Of course, this particular study took place in a very specific setting. Automatic administration of painkillers can only be done in the hospital, where a researcher can control the exact moment that pain treatment ends (unlike self-administered treatments, where patients know when they are and are not receiving treatment). Could the same effects arise in other settings? Research says yes, and this becomes clear when we take a look at something called "biosimilars."

Biosimilars are best described as cheaper alternatives to biologics—biological medical products like immune modulators, hormones, and vaccines. Doctors use biologics to treat many health conditions, including autoimmune diseases and diabetes. For instance, insulin is a biologic drug. Biologics are pretty expensive compared to conventional drugs, and many of them are still patented—meaning that their production process is a secret of the company that produces them. But when patents expire, other companies can develop biosimilars. Biosimilars have the same properties as the biologics that were originally brought onto the market. Because the patent no longer belongs to a single manufacturer, many pharmacological companies can develop and produce biosimilars. This promotes competition between companies. As a result, biosimilars are cheaper and healthcare costs can be reduced. This all may seem like a positive development. However, the cheaper price may come with a nonfinancial cost, as Dr. Bente Glintborg and her colleagues demonstrated.[8] They followed more than fifteen hundred people with inflammatory arthritis in Denmark who made the switch from biologics to biosimilars. Almost 10 percent of them stopped treatment after a few months. The main reason was that they did not feel as if the medicine was very effective. But was the biosimilar truly less effective? Not really, since the swelling and inflammation of the joints that characterize inflammatory arthritis did not change at all. Physically, the biosimilars worked just as well as the biologics did before. Instead, the perceived lack of effectiveness among the patients was exactly that: perception. Patients could have had doubts about the switch or felt anxious with the new medicine. Whatever the reason, it led them to feel like they experienced fewer positive medical effects of the biosimilar. Nocebo effects might have been at play here.

A survey among Belgian rheumatologists and their patients found that physicians were more likely than patients to express concerns about the safety, quality, and pricing of biosimilars.[9] If the negative attitude of the doctor rubs off on patients—if the doctor expresses doubts when the switch is discussed, for instance—this could impact treatment. Clearly, the doctor does not mean to evoke nocebo effects. They believe they act in the interest of the patient when expressing their doubts (e.g., "Let's not be too enthusiastic; the treatment may not work well"). But nocebo effects stand in the way of their good intentions. When doctors express doubt about the effectiveness of biosimilars, this can undermine the trust that their patients have in the treatment, causing some patients to start experiencing nocebo effects. The bad news is that many doctors do not seem to be aware of how their words can lead to nocebo effects. Would the subjective lack of effects that patients experienced from biosimilars have been different in Glintborg's study[10] if the doctors had reassured their patients that these medicines were just as effective as biologics? Perhaps. As it is, we need to increase the awareness of nocebo effects among doctors and other healthcare professionals and teach them to communicate about treatment in such a way that nocebo effects can be avoided.

We will return to the topic of what doctors can do with respect to nocebo effects in Chapter 8.

CAN WORDS HURT?

Good communication is not just important in the case of biosimilars or other drug therapies. Doctors may evoke nocebo effects unintentionally during regular medical practice. Some routine practices can be unpleasant for the patient, after all. Even if someone is not scared of needles, the sensation of a needle pricking the skin can still feel unpleasant. Can this sensation also be influenced by the nocebo effect? At Tufts Medical Center in Boston, Dr. Dirk Varelmann and his co-workers conducted a study to try to answer this question.[11] They gave one of two sets of instructions to women who needed local anesthesia before labor. They told the women either that they would "feel a big sting and burn in their back" and that "this was the worst of the procedure" or that they were going to inject "the local anesthetic" that "would make them feel comfortable during the procedure." Women who were told that the injection would feel like a big sting reported more pain from the injection than women who were told that a local anesthetic was injected. This shows that just a change in words can make a big difference.

When we see study results like those of Varelmann's team, we can speculate whether pain will always increase when we talk about it. In some ways that makes sense. When we introduce a procedure as painful, this may cause people not only to expect more pain but also to feel anxious or stressed during the procedure. These negative feelings can then exacerbate pain. From that perspective, it seems reasonable to avoid mentioning future pain as much as possible, but this is not what happens in the clinic. Healthcare professionals have good intentions, and most prefer to warn their patients that pain may be coming. "Big sting," "big ouch," and "worst part" are common descriptions by anesthetists and labor nurses, according to Varelmann,[12] and these words can sound harsh.

People do not experience nocebo effects exclusively in medical treatments and procedures, however. Sometimes the symptoms that bother them are, in fact, nocebo effects.

MIMICKING ALLERGIC SYMPTOMS

In the late nineteenth century, American medical doctor John Noland Mackenzie described the case of a female patient who was suffering from an allergy to roses, called "rose cold" at the time.[13] In an experiment, Mackenzie invited the patient for a medical consultation. Right before she arrived, Mackenzie hid an artificial rose—"of such exquisite workmanship that it presented a perfect counterfeit of the original"—in the room with the patient, but in a place where she could not see it. The conversation started normally, with Mackenzie asking how she was feeling; the patient replied that she felt fine at that moment. About halfway through the consultation, the doctor pulled out the artificial rose. Within minutes, the woman's allergy returned—she wanted to sneeze, her nose and ears were intensely itchy, her nose was congested and running, and she started to feel that she might be on the verge of an asthma attack.

This report again underlines the potential impact of negative expectancies and beliefs on how symptoms are experienced. The way the rose looked served, in this case, as a cue to which the patient responded. One possibility is that when the patient saw the artificial rose, she consciously expected symptoms to start, so much so that it induced a nocebo effect. Or, equally possible, she may have associated roses so strongly with allergic symptoms in the past that this happened automatically, outside her conscious awareness. When the doctor explained that the rose was fake, the woman obviously felt very surprised and amazed that she reacted in this way. The report then describes that she returned to the doctor's office a few days later and demonstrated that her allergic reaction to roses had disappeared completely.

One might argue that the woman with the rose is just a single case and we shouldn't read too much into it. There are many more studies that show similar situations, though. These studies provide us with further evidence that nocebo effects can trigger physiological reactions like allergies do.

The immune system also reacts to cues present in our environment and negative expectancies. This is well documented in a research paper by Maryann Gauci and her colleagues, for example.[14] They conducted an experiment in which patients with a dust mite allergy were exposed to those allergens. In one group, they combined exposure to the allergens with a milk shake of a unique color and smell. A little while later, these patients drank the same milk shake for a second time, but without exposure to dust mites. The researchers then took samples of the fluid in the patients' noses, where they measured physical signs of the allergic response such as signs of inflammation. What's important about this experiment is that the second time people drank the milk shake, their immune system reacted to it: inflammation in the nasal fluid increased. It was almost as though they had suddenly become allergic to the milk shake, too!

The same principle as in the cases of anticipatory nausea in children applies here: the body responds to cues it gets from the environment, cues signaling that something bad will happen. In this case, the cue is as innocuous as a milk shake, and the something bad is the allergic reaction.

WHERE DO WE GO FROM HERE?

As you can see, nocebo effects impact many aspects of health, medicine, and treatment. Does this mean that doctors are oblivious to the impact of the nocebo effect on their patients? Our research group recently distributed a survey to Dutch healthcare professionals, including medical doctors and nurses, to gain some insight into this question.[15] The clinicians who responded to the survey underestimated the influence of nocebo effects. Most were uncertain whether negative expectancies could even influence treatment outcomes. Only around half of them were able to give a concrete example of when they had seen an example of this in their practice. In contrast, however, most clinicians were familiar with placebo effects, and most of them did believe that positive expectancies influence treatment. But there was a blind spot when it came to negative expectancies. One of the challenges in the future is to increase awareness of nocebo effects among clinicians. This is important, as the consequences of those effects may be severe—as, for example, in the case of statins, where simply informing patients about side effects caused them to have more side effects.

Even if nocebo effects are caused by negative expectancies, this does not mean that they are merely "all in the head." Nocebo effects are just as real as regular side effects or symptoms, and people do suffer from them. Because of this, it is important that we find a way to deal with them. Research has identified some strategies to reduce nocebo effects in the clinic, which you can read more about in Chapter 8.

CHAPTER 2

WHEN PSYCHOTHERAPY HARMS

Cosima Locher and Helen Koechlin

THE DODO BIRD, THE PLACEBO EFFECT, AND PSYCHOTHERAPY

In Lewis Carroll's novel *Alice in Wonderland*, several characters needed to dry off after swimming around in Alice's pool of tears. The Dodo Bird asked them to race around the lake until they were dry. Nobody cared to measure when a competitor started to run, or how long it took them. When the characters asked the Dodo who had won the race, he thought for a long time and then replied: "Everybody has won and all must have prizes."[1]

There is an analogy between the Dodo Bird and the outcome of different psychotherapies. It's important to understand that not all psychotherapy is the same. Various psychological approaches can differ dramatically. They use different methods and tools, have different histories, and rely on different theories to explain the cause of symptoms.[2] Cognitive behavioral therapy (CBT), perhaps the technique most widely used by therapists today, assumes that the way we think about others and the world—so-called cognitive representations—influences how we respond, act, and feel. Patients

can feel better by observing and changing their thoughts and beliefs, which is possible through reflection and practice.[3]

This is very different from person-centered therapy, an approach that focuses on the patient's identity. According to the
person-centered approach, healing is achieved by living in congru-
ence, such that the patient's experiences are consistent with their
self-concept. A psychotherapist with a background in CBT might
concentrate on your thoughts and how they could become more
adaptive. A therapist who practices a person-centered approach
might try to be very empathic and to feel the resonance. Despite
these very different theories about how psychotherapy works, CBT,
person-centered, and other approaches all "win," just like all the
runners in *Alice in Wonderland*. Different therapies lead to a similar
improvement in depression, anxiety, or whatever other symptom is
being treated.[4] In other words, it doesn't matter much what type of
therapy is used. They all work equally well.

But why is this the case? Even if therapies are different from
each other, as shown in the description of CBT and person-centered
therapy, they still have important similarities. They all rely on common factors, elements that are shared across all the different methods. For example, regardless of which therapy technique a therapist
uses, they will probably form a positive and trust-based relationship with the patient, encourage positive expectations, and offer a
reasonable-sounding explanation about why their preferred therapy
approach is helpful.[5]

And as it turns out, common factors are closely related to the
placebo effect. If you swallow an inert sugar pill, its effect depends a
lot on whether you trust your physician, whether you have positive

expectations, and whether you find the explanation for taking the pill plausible. Thus, these common factors are important not only in medicine, when a patient swallows a pill, but also for every type of psychotherapy. In fact, they seem to matter even more than the tools and methods specific to the therapy.[6] This is notable, given that very different tools and methods are used in various psychotherapeutic approaches.

Let's look at a patient who is worried about failing an exam. CBT therapists might use the method of cognitive restructuring. They may focus on the patient's automatic thought "What if I fail the exam?" and will help them reflect on alternative explanations, on worst- and best-case scenarios, and so on. Therapists with a person-centered therapy approach might focus more on the therapeutic relationship—for example, "I can really see and understand that you are afraid to fail the exam. We're in this together." By being empathic and authentic, the therapist shows that they are trustworthy. It also serves as a model for patients, encouraging them to be their true selves, expressing their thoughts and feelings.

These reflections lead to a question: What exactly is the role of the counterpart to placebo, the nocebo effect in psychotherapy? Generally, and as outlined in the introduction of this book, the nocebo effect means that people are getting worse because they engage in processes that trigger specific negative expectancies (such as expecting more pain) or because they have a distrustful interaction with their physician. Both can lead to negative emotional and physical reactions on the part of patients.[7] The same holds true for psychotherapy. Negative scenarios in therapy include a patient who does not trust the therapist (for example, because the therapist is not very empathic); a patient who has negative expectations about the therapy because they had bad experiences in the past with the healthcare system or even therapy itself; and a patient who is not convinced by the explanation of why the therapy might be helpful. Although such doubts and uncertainties are surely common and to some extent normal, there is not much research into nocebo effects in psychotherapy. What's more, although psychotherapy can lead to negative consequences, such effects are regrettably underreported and underinvestigated in psychotherapy research.[8] But research in the context of psychotherapy is complex: not all negative changes in psychotherapy are necessarily due to nocebo effects, and the contributions of different factors are difficult to disentangle.[9] If, for example, a patient becomes more anxious during psychotherapy, this could be due to nocebo effects, but it could also be caused by the natural history of the disorder or a negative life event. After all, symptoms wax and wane over time for all sorts of reasons. And sometimes patients in therapy feel worse before they start to feel better.

Nocebo effects are not only a common occurrence in clinical practice but also relevant to the way in which research is conducted. This becomes apparent in the case of the waiting-list control group. When researchers aim to examine a type of psychotherapy, they often compare it with a waiting-list control group. In a waiting-list group, participants do not receive any immediate treatment, but are instead put on a waiting list to receive the psychotherapy sessions after the study is completed. Participants in the waiting-list control group often experience a worsening of symptoms.[10] This is surprising, because these patients have often lived for several years with more or less constant complaints. Thomas Baskin and colleagues argued that this might be due to nocebo effects. Participants are often disappointed to not receive the promising psychotherapeutic approach that is being tested right at the beginning of the study.[11]

Imagine that you are very afraid of spiders. You have not gone camping in years—an activity you always valued a lot—since your phobia would dominate the whole experience. You have finally worked up the courage to enroll in a psychotherapy study to treat your phobia, as you have been invited on a camping weekend by your best friends. If you were now told that you have to wait another month before you could start the therapy, you would probably be disappointed. You would miss the camping weekend, and you might decide that there is no value in facing your fears.

The previous reflections show that it can be quite challenging to detect the nocebo effect and disentangle it from other factors, both in practice and in research. You'll read more about this in Chapter 4. Nevertheless, there are some important findings about how and why nocebo effects occur in psychotherapy.

WHEN PSYCHOTHERAPY HARMS

There is probably not a single trigger that causes nocebo effects in psychotherapy. Rather, it is often an interplay of different factors that lead to a worsening of symptoms during the psychotherapeutic process. Let's use two patient cases to illustrate this.

Anna decided to start therapy after experiencing the death of her husband. She has a supportive social network and a good job that allows her to work on a flexible schedule. Anna has never been in therapy, but she has heard from friends how useful it can be.

Kate, on the other hand, has suffered from chronic depression for two years. She has made many attempts at therapy in the past and is skeptical whether a new psychotherapy approach will be more useful than the ones she has already tried. Some of Kate's clinicians were not able to help her or did not fully understand her suffering. Kate also lost her job because she could not get out of bed in the morning and function normally in daily life. Both patients will surely have different treatment expectations based on their previous experiences. Anna will be open and optimistic about psychotherapy; Kate will be rather skeptical and pessimistic.

Likewise, we know that different expectations, beliefs about illness, and beliefs about life's meaning,[12] as well as personality features such as anxiety or pessimism,[13] are relevant for the development of nocebo reactions.

Psychotherapy traditionally takes place in a one-on-one setting, and the therapist plays a crucial role when it comes to nocebo effects. Negative expectations are explainable not only by the patient's background but also by the words the therapist uses. It is not surprising that nocebo has been described as a case of "when words are painful."[14] Therapist-patient interactions that do not successfully communicate acceptance and understanding can indeed be painful for a patient. If a therapist says to Kate that she is "a high-risk patient for having depression her whole life," Kate may not feel seen in her desire for the symptoms to stop. She will probably also have the impression that the therapist has no hope for her, and so will feel even worse. It would be completely different if the therapist says that "many patients suffer from depression for years. I can support you to cope with it." While this statement also holds the uncertainty about how Kate's symptoms will develop in the future, it focuses on coping with the depression and the therapist's role in supporting Kate. In this scenario, Kate may be hopeful for the future and feel well taken care of. This will be a novel experience for her that could lead to a therapeutic change, to a process of healing.

Nocebo effects can also operate on a more subtle level. Let's go back to our example. In a session, Anna describes how sad she is since her husband died and how lonely she feels because there is now a huge hole in her life that she feels can never be filled. The therapist can feel empathy and compassion when Anna is talking about her loss, but he may say something that gives Anna the impression he trivializes her suffering,[15] such as "You do not have to worry. You will feel better in the future." This is very different from "I can understand that your loss makes you very, very sad. I do not know where your journey will lead you. But I will be on your side." Both statements have the intention of expressing hope. But they come across very differently to Anna. They convey different levels of acceptance and validation of Anna's current emotional state. In the first example, the psychotherapist may unintentionally and unconsciously trigger a nocebo effect. Anna might experience a worsening of symptoms because she might feel not taken seriously in her suffering. Of course, despite their best efforts, therapists may not always achieve the right tone. The way a message is perceived is dependent on the patient, and communication is influenced by the larger context (such as the social and cultural context of patient and therapist) as well. Hence, it is most important for therapists to be aware that words can play a powerful role in the therapeutic process and should be chosen carefully.

Patients' expectations are probably the best-established mechanism of nocebo effects. Another consideration that has gained increasing interest in recent years is the role of misattribution. As you'll hear more about in Chapter 6, misattribution can mean that a normal worsening of symptoms within the natural ebb and flow of a disorder is inappropriately attributed to a failure of psychotherapy.[16] Let's go back to our example. In the first session, the therapist informs Anna that sometimes psychotherapy can lead to unwanted outcomes. These encompass treatment failure, therapeutic risk such as the occurrence of nocebo effects, costs, and side effects.[17] As Marco Annoni will describe in Chapter 7, the therapist might be doing the right thing: from an ethical and legal perspective, it is important that therapists transparently inform their patients about the potential harms of psychotherapy.[18] In another session, Anna talks about her grief in more detail. The therapist encourages her to give her grief a *Gestalt*, to name it and describe it in more detail. Anna describes it as a black hole, which is sometimes also gray. She feels it in her chest. All energy is sucked away; her head is empty. Anna has almost no sensation in her legs and feet; they just function. She actually feels like a robot in her daily life. There is no joy. With the help of therapeutic guidance, Anna discovers that the hole she is feeling has a meaning: it helps her to remember her husband. This session was very intense for Anna, and she is exhausted afterward. Even worse, Anna now experiences her grief more acutely. She is left wondering whether this might be an unwanted effect of psychotherapy or whether the therapy is heading in the right direction.

Psychotherapy supports patients by enhancing their introspection; thus it may be new for Anna to be so aware of her emotions and to experience them in such an intense and embodied way. Perhaps en route to having her depression cured, Anna has to really feel the crushing sadness of her loss—to grieve her husband's death fully, and not run from the torment—because sometimes pain is, ironically, part of the healing process. Just like physical therapy to fix a shoulder injury can hurt on your way to strengthening the shoulder, psychotherapy can hurt on your way to strengthening your mind and attitude. Inner processes in psychotherapy are complex, and it can be challenging to disentangle nocebo effects from other effects. Did Anna come to the conclusion that the temporary, more intense feeling of sadness was beneficial for her inner process? Then we surely have no harmful effect of psychotherapy. Or did she just become more sensitive to changes in her feeling of grief because she has been made aware that psychotherapy can lead to side effects? Then we might have a case of the nocebo effect.

LABELS MATTER

So far, we have focused on patient- and physician-specific components that are related to the occurrence of nocebo effects in psychotherapy. However, there is also the more general impact of the healthcare system and the use of labels and diagnoses in the medical system. To illustrate this, consider the example of patients who suffer from chronic pain conditions where the reason for the pain is unknown. This actually occurs often for people with conditions such as chronic low back pain, irritable bowel syndrome, myalgic encephalomyelitis, and fibromyalgia. The x-rays and other tests reveal no cause, but the patient still hurts, and it is not exactly clear *why* they hurt. These chronic pain conditions should be treated not only by a medical doctor but also by a psychotherapist, since they always have both physical and mental components.[19] Some guidelines actually recommend education and psychological treatments as first-line interventions for chronic pain, before pharmacological treatment.[20] Patients who live with chronic pain conditions often share the experience of a long and unsuccessful treatment history.[21] In many cases, these patients strive to find a clear explanation for their pain and so they search for another doctor if the first one they consult cannot provide a satisfying answer—a phenomenon that has been labeled "doctor hopping" or "doctor shopping."[22] Because chronic pain is not purely a physical experience but is always linked with emotions and social consequences, patients often have appointments with medical doctors *and* psychotherapists, who might use different explanations and terms, which makes the whole issue even more confusing for patients.

Our modern medical system suggests that there is always a clear cause for a condition, something that we can treat or even eliminate as soon as we discover it. That being so, why would a patient not look for a doctor who they think will offer successful treatment? So far, chronic pain conditions without a specific cause have been called functional pain, medically unexplained pain, somatoform disorders, nonspecific pain, or psychosomatic symptoms.[23] These terms imply that for those patients, the pain might be imagined— that it might be "all in their head." Such an implication might lead to reduced compliance with medical advice and a worsening of symptoms. Here, nocebo effects work on a broader level: by giving a disease a certain label, we change the way patients (and physicians) perceive it. Along similar lines, one of the most common narratives that patients with chronic pain use is: "I am damaged and so I need a more powerful painkiller."[24] This labeling can easily evoke a nocebo effect. Patients have very low expectations in general, both of themselves and of the painkiller. They stop having hope, motivation, and a positive outlook. These attitudes all lead to the need to constantly increase the dosage—even if it is never enough.

How can such negative assumptions be changed? The introduction of a new name could be promising. The International Classification of Diseases, 11th Revision (ICD-11), created a new diagnostic entity for chronic pain, called chronic primary pain. The diagnosis of chronic primary pain can be given *independently* of identified biological or psychological contributors.[25] This shifts the focus away from the cause of a pain and acknowledges that the *pain itself* is the primary condition. One can hope that the use of a new label will enable patients to feel seen with their condition, to have the impression that their suffering is taken seriously. Time will show us more—at this point, the ICD-11 is not yet implemented in clinical practice.

Of course, another name for a condition could also influence the patient-physician interaction. With patients suffering chronic pain, physicians can find it challenging to convey the understanding that *pain itself* is the primary condition. When pain is acute, the patient needs to be supported in the understanding that the pain is a necessary and adaptive bodily function. The physician might say something like "If you avoid walking on a broken leg, you prevent further damage that additional weight bearing will inflict on your bones." In contrast, the difference between acute and chronic pain could be explained with something like "The pain sensation associated with placing your hand on a hot stove will lead to reflexive withdrawal of your hand, therefore minimizing serious burning. However, if your system remains in a constant state of alarm—that is, if pain does not fade after the initial acute phase—pain stops working very well as a way of alerting you to possible harm."[26]

Along similar lines, it has also been proposed that the use of metaphors can be helpful. A nice example comes from a research team that collaborated closely with patients and developed a joint narrative or metaphor for chronic pain.[27] In this metaphor, the body is presented as a "very, very clever computer." Patients are told that bodies, like computers, can have two kinds of problems: a hardware problem or a software problem. A hardware problem can be easily fixed; likewise, modern medicine is successful at detecting and solving hardware problems, like a broken bone. This stands in clear contrast to software problems. A software problem is hard to detect; it is usually caused by the body when patients "keep going" despite stop signals such as pain and fatigue. Chronic pain is usually a software problem. With this metaphor, patients are encouraged to actively change their body's software by adapting their lifestyle— that is, by doing things that do not create stop signals but instead enable the body to heal itself. This is a challenging task, but it shows the patient that while chronic pain conditions may never fully vanish, there is a way to actively cope with them.

The use of metaphors in the psychotherapeutic process illustrates that words can make a difference; they can generate meaning. But if not used carefully, metaphors also have the potential to harm or to mislead. They can seem like overgeneralizations, platitudes, or simplifications. A patient might feel unseen, sent off without being taken seriously. A good way to avoid a nocebo response is to ask for feedback—for example, "Is this metaphor plausible and helpful for you?" A psychotherapist can only make an offer; it is always the patient who decides whether this offer is helpful or not. As in our previous examples, it all comes back to the need to have a trust-based therapist-patient interaction that allows a shared understanding of the patient's suffering to develop.

Our examples illustrate how nocebo effects can operate in different layers of the psychotherapeutic process. They might be related to the patient's unique sociocultural background and previous life experiences, but they are also inherently linked with the physician and, most importantly, the patient-physician interaction. Notably, nocebo effects do not only occur in one-on-one settings; they are embedded in culture, as we'll cover in Chapter 12, and more specifically in the healthcare system. Here, we have outlined that labels such as "nonspecific" can indeed hurt, since patients with chronic primary pain may not feel understood and seen in their suffering. We hope that it has now become clear that words are a powerful tool in psychotherapy—unfortunately, not only in the positive direction. Clinicians should be mindful of the words they use. If a patient feels rejected or not seen, the patient can ask the therapist what exactly they meant by a specific statement. But this requires a certain level of trust. Even if patients trust their provider, they might want to avoid conflicts. Therefore, we can only encourage patients and physicians to seek a counterpart who speaks the same language. This might minimize the chances that nocebo effects occur on the therapist's couch.

CHAPTER 3

THE NOCEBO EFFECT AND COVID-19

Kate MacKrill

The United Nations described it as a "once-in-a-lifetime pandemic." As of this writing, almost three years after COVID-19 was first identified, over 600 million people worldwide have been infected with the disease and millions have died from it. The pandemic has resulted in marked changes to our normal lives and the functioning of society. People adapted to wearing face masks (previously uncommon outside of a few Asian countries), social distancing, lockdowns, and travel restrictions, among other challenges. Vaccination was heralded as a key strategy in combating COVID-19 and allowing societies to return to a new normal. However, even before the pandemic, hesitancy about being vaccinated was common and often fueled by concerns about side effects.[1] The development of several effective vaccines against COVID-19 was met with some concerns about the long-term safety of the vaccines.[2] The COVID-19 pandemic and the global vaccination campaigns provided a perfect environment for the nocebo effect.

***

THE NOCEBO EFFECT FROM THE VACCINE

Like many medical treatments, people receiving the COVID-19 vaccine are susceptible to the nocebo effect due to negative expectations about vaccine side effects. The first telltale signs of nocebo response came from the initial trials testing the efficacy and safety of the newly developed vaccine. In these vaccine trials, one group of participants received the real COVID-19 vaccine, while another group was injected with saline—a substance that does not have any effect on the body and is used as a placebo control. To determine whether the vaccine protected people against the virus, researchers then compared how many participants from the two groups went on to contract COVID-19. Another important aim of the clinical trials was to establish the safety of the vaccine. To do this, the researchers also examined differences in side effect reporting to see if there were any negative symptoms reported at higher rates in the vaccine group compared to the placebo group.

When these studies were published, additional researchers were able to combine the results of many different vaccine trials to produce a more complete picture of how likely side effects were from the COVID-19 vaccine. Three of these bigger studies (also called reviews) combining results from smaller experiments were published in January 2022. They looked at the rate of adverse reaction reporting in the placebo groups of COVID-19 vaccine trials.[3] While the rate of side effects was higher in the real vaccine groups, as would be expected, all three reviews found a large overlap in the types of side effects reported by participants who received the actual vaccine and those who received the placebo injection of saline. For example, the review by Dr. Martina Amanzio and colleagues found that while around 55 percent of those receiving the active vaccine reported a general adverse reaction, the most common symptoms being headaches and fatigue, 42 percent of the placebo group also reported these general symptoms.[4] Similarly, the review by Dr. Julia Haas and colleagues reported that after one dose, 46 percent of participants who received the vaccine reported at least one general adverse reaction, and 35 percent of the placebo group also reported a general side effect. This suggests that a large proportion of side effects cannot be attributed to the vaccine. In fact, one review estimated that the nocebo effect could account for 76 percent of the side effects from the COVID-19 vaccine.[5]

In addition to clinical trials, studies conducted during the rollout of the COVID-19 vaccine to the general public also provide evidence for the role of negative expectations in producing side effects. In one study, participants completed a questionnaire measuring various psychological variables prior to receiving the vaccine, such as worry about COVID-19, expectations for experiencing side effects from the vaccine, perceived sensitivity to medicines, and depression. Of all the factors, expecting to experience an adverse reaction was most strongly associated with experiencing side effects later.[6] In a similar study, the more hesitant people felt about having the second vaccine dose, the more side effects they reported after the booster shot six months later.[7] These findings may be due to the nocebo effect, but it might also be that people who genuinely react more to the active ingredient in vaccines feel more hesitant about being vaccinated. However, research has shown that believing you are sensitive to the effects of medicines means you do experience more side effects, even from a placebo tablet.[8]

Researchers have examined the impact of COVID-19 policies on side effect reporting, in particular the move from voluntary vaccination to it being a mandatory requirement for social engagement, as happened in some countries. It is thought that a lack of personal choice could increase vaccine hesitancy and side effect concerns, thereby exacerbating the nocebo effect. This was the case when France introduced a vaccine mandate requiring members of the public to be double vaccinated in order to enter certain public spaces, such as cafes and shops. The proportion of people reporting side effects from the vaccine increased from 34 percent prior to the mandate to 57 percent after it was implemented, suggesting that feeling pressured to be vaccinated can contribute to nocebo effects.[9] Due to our ever-evolving understanding of COVID-19 and the vaccines, some of the trends seen are likely to be a result of the nocebo effect and some may be from other causes.

THE MEDIA AND THE NOCEBO EFFECT

The word "unprecedented" has been frequently used to describe the COVID-19 pandemic. People have found themselves trying to function in an uncertain and ever-changing environment, and the media has played a significant beneficial role with its ability to communicate public health information rapidly to a wide audience. However, the media also mirrors public reaction and anxiety, which has been reflected in dramatic and negative information about the pandemic on news and social media.[10] In discussing COVID-19 vaccination, the media focused heavily on rare side effects, such as blood clots from the AstraZeneca vaccine (which have a 0.0004 percent chance of occurring) or myocarditis from the Pfizer vaccine

(0.003 percent chance). Such media coverage increased the public's worry about vaccine side effects.[11] This attention on side effects can impact people's negative expectations and exacerbate the nocebo effect from the COVID-19 vaccine, as was the case in New Zealand.

On August 30, 2021, the New Zealand government's Ministry of Health released a statement that a woman had died after receiving the Pfizer COVID-19 vaccine. The death was attributed to the rare side effect myocarditis, an inflammation of the heart wall that is characterized by chest pain, shortness of breath, and an abnormal heartbeat. New Zealand print, television, and radio media platforms discussed this case and encouraged people to be vigilant for cardiac symptoms following vaccination. There were two further deaths in New Zealand from myocarditis, one in December 2021 and another in April 2022, which again received substantial media attention. While myocarditis is a serious side effect of the Pfizer COVID-19 vaccine, it is rare. A study from Israel found that 2.7 people per 100,000 vaccinated experienced myocarditis following the Pfizer vaccine.[12] However, the symptoms of myocarditis, such as chest pain and shortness of breath, are not uncommon in the general population. Population surveys show that in an average week, around 13 percent of people experience breathing problems and 7 percent experience chest pain and 7 percent experience heart palpitations that cannot be attributed to a particular cause.[13] Consequently, media attention on myocarditis and its symptoms might cause people to overestimate its prevalence, resulting in them misattributing everyday symptoms to the vaccine and reporting them as side effects. You'll learn more about misattribution in Chapters 4 and 6.

In my research as a health psychologist, I have investigated the effect mainstream media coverage can have in exacerbating the nocebo effect. Later in the book, I'll explore the power of the media in more detail (see Chapter 11), but when it comes to COVID-19 vaccinations, we can also draw out connections. The case of the New Zealand media linking myocarditis to the COVID-19 vaccine seemed to me like a prime situation for the nocebo effect to occur. Using publicly available data on vaccine side effects reported to the New Zealand Centre for Adverse Reaction Monitoring (CARM), I investigated whether the reporting of the three symptoms mentioned in the media (chest discomfort, breathing problems, and altered heart rate) increased following the media coverage.[14] I looked at the reporting rates per 100,000 vaccinations in the seven months prior to the news coverage on myocarditis, and compared this with the reporting rate in the nine months after the first news item in August 2021.

Prior to the media attention on vaccine-induced myocarditis, CARM received an average of 35 reports of chest pain per 100,000 vaccinations. After the media coverage, this increased considerably, to 220 reports. A similar change was seen for breathing problems, which went from 25 to 113 reports, and for heart rhythm symptoms, which increased from 34 to 133 reports. To provide further evidence that it was the media's focus on these particular side effects that was responsible for this change, I also examined the reporting rate of three control side effects that had not received media attention: musculoskeletal pain, numbness, and fever. The reporting of these side effects did not change that much. For example, musculoskeletal pain went from 41 reports per 100,000 vaccinations before the coverage to 52 reports after.

The symptoms of myocarditis mentioned in the media are also common symptoms of anxiety. It is possible that news stories on deaths attributed to myocarditis provoked concerns about the safety of the vaccine, with the symptoms of chest pain, heart rate, and breathing problems attributed to the vaccine being due to anxiety instead. Prior to the alarmist media coverage, CARM received an average of 15 reports of anxiety per 100,000 vaccinations, which increased to 73 reports following the news items. What's more, statistical analyses showed that the experience of anxiety was significantly associated with greater attribution of chest pain, breathing problems, and changes in heart rate to the vaccine. This shows that anxiety was responsible for some of the increase in side effects.

In addition to the individual symptoms, the actual cardiac condition myocarditis could be reported to CARM. Prior to the media coverage, myocarditis had an average rate of 0.6 reports per 100,000 vaccinations. After the media coverage described this condition and linked it to the Pfizer COVID-19 vaccine, the reporting rate increased to 11 per 100,000. While 11 as a total number might sound small, it represents an increase of 1,700 percent. This significant increase in myocarditis could be a genuine vaccine response, or it might be due to self-diagnosis. Anyone in New Zealand can submit a medicine adverse reaction report to CARM. Community doctors typically submit around 65 percent of reports, but in the case of the COVID-19 vaccine, they were responsible for only 13 percent. This suggests that a large number of reports of myocarditis came directly from members of the public, who may have interpreted their chest or breathing symptoms as being myocarditis rather than considering other explanations, such as anxiety.

Taken together, these results suggest that a nocebo effect did occur following the media attention on vaccine-induced myocarditis. It is likely that the media coverage, which discussed a death linked to the vaccine and the symptoms of myocarditis, influenced people's expectations for side effects, prompted greater attention to symptoms, and led to the misattribution of these to the vaccine. These symptoms are frequently experienced in the general population, and it is possible that media attention influenced people's perceptions and attribution of these common symptoms. This is supported by the fact that the symptoms the media specifically warned about (chest pain, breathing problems, and heart rate changes) saw a sudden increase in reports to CARM, while side effects that did not receive media attention did not see a substantial change in the number of reports. The changes in the cardiac and breathing symptoms could be due to increased anxiety, as concerns about COVID-19 have already been shown to be associated with experiencing a greater number of unexplained physical symptoms.[15]

THE NOCEBO EFFECT AND COVID-19 SYMPTOMS

Not only are vaccine side effects impacted by the nocebo effect, but the actual symptoms of COVID-19 can be as well. If you have the characteristic symptoms of COVID-19, such as a sore throat, fever, or tiredness, it must be because you actually have COVID-19, right? But what if you only have those symptoms because you *think* you have COVID? A large study from France investigated whether the belief that one has had COVID-19, either accurate or inaccurate, was associated with the experience of symptoms.[16] Between December 2020 and January 2021, participants in the study were asked whether they believed they had previously been infected by the coronavirus. They were asked to identify any ongoing symptoms they were experiencing from a list of twenty, such as headache, sleep problems, dizziness, heart palpitations, and cough. Participants also provided a blood sample to detect SARS-CoV-2 antibodies, which would confirm a previous COVID-19 infection.

The study was conducted in the early stages of the pandemic and involved more than 26,000 participants, of whom only 1,091 had a positive blood test confirming a past COVID-19 infection. However, irrespective of whether a person had previously had COVID-19 according to the blood test, it was the belief in having been infected that was more strongly associated with the experience of ongoing symptoms. For example, of the participants who returned a positive blood test and *believed* they'd had COVID, 14 percent reported ongoing fatigue. This is compared to only 4 percent of people who did not believe they'd had COVID despite having a positive blood test. Similarly, fatigue was reported by 13 percent of people who believed they'd had COVID even though their blood test showed they were never infected, compared to 3 percent who had a negative blood test and correctly believed that they'd not had COVID. Put another way, while you're two and a half times more likely to experience fatigue if you've actually had COVID than if you've never had it, you're five times more likely to have fatigue if you *think* you've had it.

Further research provides evidence for the role of beliefs and expectations in the manifestation of COVID-19 symptoms. Despite not having a positive COVID-19 test, people who were nevertheless certain that they had COVID experienced more severe symptoms.[17]

A similar study, led by Dr. Liron Rozenkrantz at Bar-Ilan University in Israel, found that the more severe someone believed their symptoms would be if they contracted COVID-19, the greater the number of COVID-like symptoms they experienced several weeks later.[18] These results suggest that particular expectations about COVID-19, such as it being a severe illness or merely thinking that we have contracted it, may influence our later symptoms. These expectations could make us more likely to pay attention to our body, be on the alert for characteristic symptoms, and potentially misattribute these to the illness.

It is also worth discussing the role of misinformation and conspiracy theories in shaping negative expectations about the COVID-19 pandemic and having an adverse effect on health. Misinformation and conspiracies about COVID-19 and the vaccines have been rife throughout the pandemic, in particular via social media. Conspiracies can include beliefs that the virus is a biological weapon, that it is a hoax, and that the vaccine contains microchips to control the population. Believing in COVID-19 conspiracies results in being less likely to physically distance, wear face masks, or be vaccinated.[19] Conspiracy theorists also experience more anxiety, depression, and feelings of powerlessness. This could be considered another consequence of the nocebo effect and the impact of our negative expectations on our well-being.

REDUCING COVID-19 VACCINE NOCEBO EFFECTS

It is essential that we protect ourselves from COVID-19 to reduce our chances of ill health. Likewise, we also need to protect ourselves from the nocebo effect and the exacerbation of symptoms and side effects. Like all medical treatments, the various COVID-19 vaccines will have side effects. For the mild side effects, such as fatigue and headache, it is important to keep in mind that these are symptoms we often experience in our everyday lives and so they might not necessarily be due to the vaccine. Alternatively, if you do happen to notice symptoms after vaccination, this experience can be reframed as a sign that the vaccine is working and your body is developing immunity to COVID-19. This simple change in mindset, brought about by highlighting how side effects can be a positive sign, can mitigate the amplifying effect of anxiety and can reduce the severity of treatment-related symptoms.[20]

Another thing to remember is that the mainstream news media is motivated to report stories that will grab our attention. The COVID-19 pandemic and the vaccine have provided a wealth of such stories. It is the sensational stories about serious side effect experiences that are often discussed in the media, such as myocarditis from the Pfizer vaccine or blood clots from the AstraZeneca vaccine. While it is important to be aware of the risks associated with any treatment, these serious side effects are rare; however, repeated exposure to them through media articles can make us overestimate how prevalent they are. While it is unlikely that we will actually experience myocarditis or blood clots, these media stories increase our risk of unnecessarily experiencing other symptoms, as they elevate our expectations for side effects. While we don't have to be statisticians, we can counter this by briefly considering that the likelihood of a particular side effect is potentially far lower than the impression the news article gives. For example, the *Guardian* reported on 220 cases of blood clots following the AstraZeneca vaccine. This sounds alarming, but large-scale studies show that this side effect occurs in 1 per 250,000 people vaccinated, which is a risk of 0.0004 percent.[21] Additionally, we should remind ourselves that these side effects of the vaccine are likely far milder or even less common than the actual effects of the disease. Myocarditis is six times more likely to occur after COVID-19 infection than after vaccination.[22] Ensuring that our expectations are kept in perspective might just help immunize us against the nocebo effect.

PART TWO

HOW THE NOCEBO EFFECT WORKS

CHAPTER 4

WHAT IS THE NOCEBO EFFECT? A PHILOSOPHICAL PERSPECTIVE

Charlotte Blease

Many a small thing has been made large by the right kind of advertising.

—Mark Twain

"The Nocebo Effect: Can Our Thoughts Kill Us?" asked a compelling headline in 2015 in the *Sydney Morning Herald*. The accompanying story recounted "a distressing incident that led to a man's death in the 1700s."[1] In that incident, "students played a nasty prank on their medical professor's disliked assistant. Intending to give him a fright, they kidnapped him, telling him they were going to decapitate him. They blindfolded him, laid his head on a chopping block and draped a wet cloth over his neck. Convinced he was about to die, the assistant died instantly." What was the purported cause? None other than the nocebo effect, we are told.

In the same year the article ran, 2015, Gizmodo, a popular science website, ran another horror story, about a young man who was hospitalized for swallowing sugar pills.[2] According to anecdotal reports, the man—who was being treated for depression—swallowed an entire bottle of "medication" in a suicide attempt after his girlfriend dumped him. Realizing he wanted to live, the young man immediately admitted himself to the hospital, where, we are told, "grievously ill, he lingered near death. He couldn't breathe. His blood pressure was dangerously low." Doctors then realized the man had been a participant in a study for a new antidepressant. But he'd been allocated to the placebo arm. It was not the poisons of a drug that led to his near-lethal illness; it was—the journalist claimed—the nocebo effect: "Convinced he was dying, he actually began to die."

Undoubtedly, these episodes make for compelling column inches and sensational stories, and as journalists say, "if it bleeds, it leads." Nor are such scoops wholly new. "Voodoo death" has also been attributed to the nocebo effect. The term was coined by physician Walter Cannon in 1942 to refer to cases in which people died within days of local traditional healers placing ritual curses on them.[3]

Aside from near-deaths and actual fatalities, the nocebo effect has been charged with causing a wide variety of troubling ailments and symptoms, as discussed throughout this book—exacerbating the side effects of medications, causing harm through overdiagnosis or overtreatment, ascribing negative health effects to wind turbines, and driving a surge in gluten intolerance, to take several examples.

What should we make of the idea that such diverse phenomena can be attributed to a single cause? On the one hand, the suggestion is both intriguing and seductive. On the other hand, some readers may already be skeptical, suspecting that if the nocebo effect explains too much, then perhaps it explains nothing at all.

One place to begin is with how we define nocebo effects. Throughout this book, contributions draw on a variety of perspectives, including from clinicians and researchers working in psychology, neurobiology, and ethics. Each offers a slightly different interpretation of nocebo phenomena. This variety is to be expected, especially when scholars from different disciplines attempt to grapple with a relatively new field. My own background is philosophy, which might seem a peculiar discipline to offer any scientific insight. However, philosophy can function as a handmaiden to science: philosophy and empirical research can be mutually enriching. In this chapter I invite you on a philosophical exploration to ask what nocebo effects might be, including, crucially, what they might *not* be.

MEDICAL SCIENCE NEEDS MARIE KONDO

Acting like Marie Kondo—the Netflix sensation who encouraged people to declutter, tidy up, and reorganize—philosophy can help us begin to put the "nocebo house" in order. It can ensure that messy or vague definitions are not swept under the carpet. To see how, and to begin the process, we need to start by understanding placebo concepts, which will also serve as a crucial cautionary tale. The nocebo effect is often characterized as the malevolent twin of the placebo effect—the yin to the placebo effect's yang (on which more shortly). Moreover, since there is comparatively limited research into the nocebo effect, placebo studies present opportunities to learn from, and even avoid, some of the challenges associated with defining these concepts: doing so will help us better understand how to define nocebo phenomena. A note of caution is in order: when it comes to placebo concepts, even mild-mannered Marie Kondo might become a little impatient at the clutter and confusion.

Consider first the term "placebo." Some clinicians and researchers assume placebos are just sugar pills or saline solutions offered to patients. Others argue placebos are treatments that have no "specific" effect on a condition or symptoms. Yet others claim placebos are any treatment given to administer hope and/or any intervention prescribed to placate—or even to get rid of—patients, especially those for whom medicine has very little to offer. Still others emphasize placebos as methodological tools used by researchers for measuring the effectiveness of treatments, and which as such are "inert" treatments. Some say placebos can be all of the above.

When it comes to the term "placebo effects," some clinicians and researchers assume this refers to the outcome of patients receiving a placebo, whether in a clinical trial or in a clinical setting. Others call these outcomes the "placebo response." While it sounds like splitting hairs, some differentiate between the terms "placebo effect" and "placebo response," arguing that "placebo effect" refers only to a positive health outcome that arises from a distinct psychobiological process or processes. Relatedly, others argue placebos are neither necessary nor sufficient to elicit placebo effects/responses.

Like someone walking into a room laden with too much clutter, readers may already be irked by the definitional disarray. Making matters worse, scientists sometimes wave their hands in the air, dismissing the idea there is a mess that needs to be sorted out. At the other extreme, researchers with a philosophical bent—Andrew

Turner among them—urge that we should eliminate the terms "placebo," "placebo response," and "placebo effect" altogether. Turner argues these terms have become so unbearably messy and confused we really need to ditch the lot and start again from scratch. The temptation may be to give in to the mess, or merely to assume that underneath it all scientists have everything in order. But there are downstream effects of giving short shrift to definitional issues, no matter how tedious the concern might initially appear. Messiness can lead to problems, and placebo studies are not without critics. For example, Oxford University philosopher and expert in the placebo effect Jeremy Howick has argued there is a risk of both underestimating and overestimating treatment effect sizes when researchers are not careful about how they conceive of placebos in clinical trials.[4] Other leading medical researchers—most of whom work outside the field of placebo studies and therefore have fewer intellectual allegiances to it—question the reliability of some well-cited findings about the size of placebo effects and the appropriateness of methodologies aimed at determining these effects.[5] In summary, future-proofing nocebo studies could help prevent similar questions about the credibility of the science from arising.

PLACEBOS AND NOCEBOS

Philosophy is not just about finger-wagging; it is about offering constructive analyses, too. Having spent more than a decade, on and off, attempting to categorize, organize, and tidy up in this field—aspiring to be the equivalent of a medical Marie Kondo—I would be remiss not to offer my own definitions of "placebo" and describe how we can use them to advance our understanding of nocebo phenomena.[6] This is not to say these interpretations are the final word on the matter. Still, what follows is a brief overview of my own attempts at systematizing and organizing.

First, consider the term "placebo." This term camouflages two very distinct clusters of meanings. In *clinical contexts*—such as when you visit the doctor—you might be offered a placebo: an intervention that is ineffective for a condition or set of symptoms but is nonetheless administered as if it was effective. In focus group research with primary care physicians, conducted with my colleague Michael Bernstein, we learned that doctors sometimes knowingly prescribe placebos. They may do this to placate patients (in fact, "placebo" is Latin for "I shall please") or even get rid of them, to elicit positive effects (potentially, "placebo effects," on which more later), or to keep up appearances as doctors, especially if they have nothing else to offer.[7] As one participant told us, "It gets done all the time." Surveys show placebo prescribing is common. In 2018, a systematic review and meta-analysis of surveys from thirteen countries found that placebos were used by 53 to 89 percent of physicians at least monthly.[8] Patients who are suffering with chronic pain, fatigue, fibromyalgia, or medically unexplained symptoms are more likely to be prescribed placebos.

The second use for the term "placebo" is very different. It refers to *clinical trials*, where investigators use study controls to establish the effectiveness of a novel drug. In randomized controlled trials, participants may be allocated to receive the real treatment or a placebo. Ideally, participants and researchers should not be able to guess whether recruits received the drug or placebo—and if they do so, this is referred to as "breaking blind." How the treatment is delivered by clinician-researchers can subtly offer hints and clues about whether the patient received a placebo or the real treatment, as can the nature of the treatment itself. To avoid this happening, both researchers and patients should be unaware of what the patient is receiving. The placebo should be indistinguishable from the specific treatment being investigated—if the treatment is a drug delivered in a tablet that is green and round, with an acidic flavor, then ideally the placebo should be designed, as far as possible, to mimic the appearance, taste, and smell of the tablet containing the real drug. The only difference is that the placebo does not have the active drug ingredient. A medicine delivered in a tablet contains the active ingredient, as you would expect, but it also contains inactive substances, called excipients. Examples include lubricants, so that the tablet does not get stuck to the machine pressing the tablet; a bulking agent, to make the tablet larger; and a disintegrant, to aid breakdown of the tablet after it is ingested by the patient. All this is quite convenient because we can create a placebo tablet, capsule, or cream by leaving out only the active ingredient.

There are lessons here for how we think about nocebo. First, just because there is a term "placebo" does not mean we need a new stand-alone term "nocebo." There is no equivalent of nocebo in clinical contexts—no clinician will deliberately give a nocebo to make patients feel worse. Nor is there an equivalent in clinical trials: placebos in this context should refer to "treatment controls," and so the idea of a nocebo control makes no sense. Therefore, when we hear or read about the singular term "nocebo," even if it is used casually or loosely, we should be wary, and we might inquire further about what is meant by it.

PLACEBO EFFECTS AND NOCEBO EFFECTS

The fuller term "nocebo effects" is meaningful, but homing in on it requires more background about placebo effects. This is the phenomenon you may have read about in newspapers or watched science reports about on TV. Placebo effects are the subject of considerable research and are increasingly recognized as genuinely salubrious effects that arise via patients' expectations about a treatment and perceptions that it might work. As a result of psychobiological mechanisms, anticipating the benefits—for example, pain relief—of a treatment in some limited circumstances can induce positive health changes, actually reducing pain. Or anticipating feeling less fatigued may, via expectancies, actually reduce tiredness. In short, placebo effects refer to health benefits caused by the expectation that an intervention will be beneficial. These expectancies may be enhanced by patient-clinician interactions or by social conventions associated with treatments, such as the custom of swallowing pills.

Mirroring placebo effects, we might define nocebo effects as arising from negative expectations (such as anticipating more pain) and, as a consequence, resulting in adverse health outcomes (namely, experiencing more pain). Studies show that increased awareness about the side effects of medications, the negative framing of information, and the low quality of interactions with clinicians can increase the risk of nocebo effects. Acting like "negative" placebo effects, then, nocebo effects are participants' negative expectations that are self-fulfilling.

Fascinating studies—albeit fewer in number than those focusing on placebo effects—show that negative health changes can arise as a result of particular negative anticipations associated with medical treatments. In his book *Placebo Effects: Understanding the Mechanisms of Health and Disease*, Italian physiologist and neuroscientist Fabrizio Benedetti reviews studies whereby patients undergoing cancer chemotherapy begin to experience nausea and vomiting before treatment, sometimes when they smell the odors of the clinic.[9] Like the famous study of Pavlov's dogs, which learned to associate the ringing of a bell with food and later salivated when the bell rang even though no food arrived, patients appeared to be similarly "conditioned" to expect to feel ill when associating the clinic environment with the adverse effects of chemotherapy.

DIFFERENTIATING NOCEBO
EFFECTS FROM OTHER NOISE

Yet sometimes we might overestimate the risk of nocebo effects. To see how this can happen, let's return to the role of placebos in clinical trials. We learned that placebos in clinical trials cannot merely be understood as "saline solutions" or "sugar pills" but should be adapted to mimic the particular intervention under scrutiny. This last point is important in trials of physical, psychological, and surgical therapies because these are complex therapies delivered within an elaborate therapeutic ritual, and deciding what aspect of the encounter is the active ingredient can be challenging. Implementing suitable placebos in clinical trials is not always easy. When placebos are successfully implemented as a control in a trial, it becomes harder for patients, clinicians, and trial staff to guess which arm of the trial a patient has been allocated to.

Why should researchers go to such lengths? The use of robust placebo controls is essential to minimize the "noise" arising in clinical trials, which interferes with accurate assessment of the effectiveness of the novel treatment under scrutiny. Here are some examples of this noise and why controls are necessary. Diseases have a "natural history" (how the disease progresses over time in an individual in the absence of treatment), and in some cases patients might get better anyway. People also respond differently when aware they're part of a research study (a reaction called the "Hawthorne effect"), and sometimes they change their behavior in positive ways when they're being monitored, which can lead to different health outcomes. Another well-established problem is that participants sometimes unintentionally report inaccurate outcomes, perhaps subconsciously attempting to please the investigator (called "response bias"). For example, if informed that the treatment will lead to better outcomes, some patients may falsely, though unwittingly, report health benefits. Yet another source of noise in clinical trials is the potential for placebo effects—positive health changes that can arise via psychological expectations.

Taken together, all of these factors—natural history, Hawthorne effect, response bias, placebo effects—are increasingly referred to as the "placebo response," capturing the outcomes that arise after, *but not necessarily because of,* receiving a placebo or a treatment. If a treatment is effective, participants in the treatment arm will experience clinically significant improvement compared with those allocated to the placebo. And if there is a placebo effect, participants in both the placebo group and the treatment group may experience better clinical outcomes than participants allocated to a no-treatment or wait-list group. Complicating matters further, even participants in no-treatment groups might report positive health changes due to the Hawthorne effect and response bias, since they too are enrolled in a trial.

If the term "placebo response" captures all the undifferentiated *positive* outcomes that arise after participants are allocated to the placebo arm in a clinical trial, using the term "nocebo response" could usefully refer to the undifferentiated *negative* outcomes that arise after receiving a placebo. Again, this could include natural history—that is, some people may feel worse, regardless of whether or not they participated in the trial. Normal life events will serve up different responses: we all have random aches and pains at times. Moreover, asking participants to focus their attention on how they feel might even increase vigilance about a variety of underlying low-level somatic complaints, as discussed by John Kelley in Chapter 6. Although the possibility has not been explored, some people might also report worse outcomes due to what we might call a negative Hawthorne effect—namely, changing their behavior in ways that lead to adverse effects on their health. For example, a researcher sets out to study diet. Some people may display a positive Hawthorne effect, where they will start to be self-conscious about eating pizza and instead eat salads. But on the other hand, some people may get stressed out about having their diet observed, throw caution to the wind, and start eating whatever they want. Response biases might also influence reported outcomes in negative ways. For example, if participants are informed about a long list of potential side effects of a treatment in a clinical trial, they might unintentionally, but falsely, report an increase in adverse effects. And finally, participants might also experience genuine nocebo effects. Differentiating genuine nocebo effects from the rest of this noise will not be an easy task.

Many researchers, clinicians, and patients strongly believe placebos have powerful clinical effects. However, as this brief tour shows, this is a methodologically complex area of study requiring a great deal of ingenuity to ensure that genuine placebo effects are measured and not overestimated. Similarly, negative outcomes following the administration of a placebo or a treatment in a clinical trial may be due to an undifferentiated amalgam of nocebo effects. Akin to differentiating placebo effects, estimating whenever genuine nocebo effects have arisen will be tricky.

AVOIDING CATEGORY MISTAKES

Using these definitions, we can now examine a variety of cases to ask whether it is reasonable to surmise nocebo effects have arisen or whether the label doesn't quite fit. Other chapters in this book will examine the relationship between treatment side effects and nocebo effects. As the foregoing discussion indicates, it is important to ask whether clinical trials can adequately differentiate nocebo effects from wider reporting about negative outcomes—what I have dubbed the "nocebo response." For example, in the recent highly publicized studies described by Kate MacKrill in Chapter 3, investigators reported that up to two-thirds of side effects of COVID-19 vaccines—such as headaches, fatigue, and malaise—were caused by the "nocebo effect" or what investigators and journalists sometimes interchangeably called the "nocebo response." In their usage, the terms appeared synonymous, both denoting the phenomenon of negative expectations causing nasty side effects. However, it is unclear whether adverse effects were directly triggered as a result of negative anticipation of vaccine side effects or whether something else was happening. For example, people recruited into the vaccine trials may have been subject to a special kind of Hawthorne effect—namely, heightened vigilance about underlying everyday somatic ailments. Another concern is responder biases, where, having been informed about potential side effects, patients might have unknowingly biased their responses. Or they may have experienced genuine nocebo effects. In short, getting clear on what we really mean by "nocebo effects" matters.

Another potential source of conceptual confusion is the claim that harms from overdiagnosis and overtreatment constitute nocebo effects. In his book *The Nocebo Effect: Overtreatment and Its Costs*,[10] Dr. Stewart Justman, of the University of Montana, argues that the overmedicalization of normal, everyday complaints—driven by Big Pharma—has led to real harms, via the side effects of drugs and unnecessary treatments, which he labels "nocebo effects." Convincing people they may have a real health problem requiring treatment, when alternatively the condition could be managed with watchful waiting, may elicit anxiety. It may also lead to a cascade of harms from overmedication or even unnecessary surgery. For example, older men with benign prostatic hyperplasia (BPH) commonly report waking up in the night needing to pee more. Around 90 percent of men in their seventies and eighties experience BPH. But treating the condition via surgery can render patients worse off, resulting in greater risk of urinary tract infections, incontinence, and sexual dysfunction. Patients can experience worse health as a result of the surgery than if nothing were done. Justman raises many important ethical concerns about overdiagnosis and overtreatment in modern medicine. However, I argue that describing these kinds of harms as "nocebo effects" in this instance is a category mistake. This is because the negative effects Justman describes are not induced by patients' anticipations but are either the result of heightened anxiety or harms resulting from injuries and impairments following unnecessary medical interventions.

Nocebo effects are also blamed for the rise of gluten sensitivity, with the idea that if people read too much negative press about gluten, they may develop sensitivity to it.[11] Again, we might wonder whether this is a case of genuine gluten intolerance or of reporters being gluttons for nocebo effects. When we take a closer look, a variety of explanations is possible. First, if indeed there is genuine increased prevalence, this might be due to greater awareness of gluten sensitivity, or changes in diet, or some other kind of environmental exposure over time. It is reasonable to explore the most obvious explanations before plumbing for the most exotic ones, like the nocebo effect. Consider the possibility that increased prevalence of gluten intolerance may be the result of better public awareness. In a survey by the Pew Internet and American Life Project conducted in 2013, 80 percent of internet users, a total of 93 million Americans, used the web to search for health information—figures that are undoubtedly higher today.[12] Among its findings is that two out of three people searching for health information online reported seeking information on specific diseases or medical issues. Roughly half searched for information about particular treatments or procedures, and around 40 percent hunted for advice about diet, nutrition, and vitamins. It is certainly possible that many of these people are better informed and simply doing a better job of self-diagnosing their gluten intolerance or bringing it to the awareness of their doctor.

On the flip side, higher rates of reporting might also be due to people misattributing ailments they already experience that are independent of gluten exposure. Or, misattributing low-level symptoms that they already experience might induce further anxieties or worries that worsen their symptoms. But even here, it is still unclear whether these symptoms constitute nocebo effects. Another explanation is also possible: because of what they've read on the internet, some people may be mistaken in their self-diagnosis—an error that is especially justifiable since there are no agreed-upon diagnostic tests for gluten sensitivity. Moreover, with an estimated seven thousand rare diseases in the world (a figure that reflects only those medicine knows about), it is possible that some patients, or indeed clinicians, might make diagnostic mistakes by attributing gastrointestinal ailments to gluten sensitivity or vice versa. Some clinicians might also incorrectly attribute gluten intolerance to mental illness—a process known as diagnostic overshadowing, which happens when reports of physical symptoms are wrongly attributed to psychiatric conditions. That is, could the condition instead be the result of a rare disease or an as yet unknown condition? Alternatively, increased rates might be a result of new dietary or environmental triggers causing genuine gluten intolerance.

It is possible that people experience gluten intolerance as a result of genuine nocebo effects, of the sort documented by Benedetti. Recall this is the idea that people anticipate gluten sensitivity and as a result of psychobiological mechanisms this anticipation becomes a self-fulfilling prophecy. There may be multiple reasons we see increased reporting of gluten sensitivity, and many explanations are unrelated to nocebo effects. Therefore, it would be useful for experimentalists to try to probe more closely the relationship between gluten sensitivity and nocebo effects.

Taking Stock Again

Tidying is often a headache, but as nocebo study develops, we will need to be ruthless in the decluttering process and decide what definitions we can justifiably keep and what is of little use. During the early emergence of novel fields of inquiry—as we have seen in these examples—researchers often talk at cross-purposes, often without even realizing it. According to philosopher and historian of science Thomas Kuhn, science doesn't truly get under way until we have settled disputes about basics, such as how a phenomenon is defined and the appropriate methods and techniques for investigating it.[13] Only when theoretical and conceptual matters are resolved, Kuhn observed, can researchers efficiently get on with the work of experimentation and what he dubbed "normal science." This includes all the activities that scientists pursue when embarking on programs of research, whether working at the lab bench, devising experiments, or conducting research out in the field. Since the field of nocebo studies is still relatively nascent—though growing—we can therefore expect some scientists and researchers, including those in this book, to adopt slightly different interpretations of the "nocebo effect" or "nocebo response." Again, this is normal.

Nonetheless, definitions can sometimes go awry for other reasons—and aspects of modern academe must shoulder some blame. Lack of clarity about terms provides fertile ground for exaggerated reporting, albeit unintentional. Scientists invest huge amounts of time in their work, which understandably fosters allegiance to pet theories and ideas. And because scientists' careers rely heavily on limited pots of national and institutional funding for which competition is fierce, the prevailing grant culture can subtly, unwittingly, incline researchers to lose important nuance. This constellation of factors means shade and subtlety can sometimes unintentionally get lost when scientists pitch proposals. As the late psychologist Dr. Scott Lilienfeld, of Emory University in Atlanta, cautioned, researchers often promise more than they deliver, and there is less time to go slow and "think deeply." The situation is made worse because funding agencies tend to make awards for big, bold research, including studies that are newsworthy or are "sold" as impacting the public.[14] Going even further, Lilienfeld warned, "In today's academic environment, big picture thinkers may be at risk for extinction." Philosophy is the ultimate big-picture discipline. So philosophers, and indeed philosophically oriented scientists, might usefully help curb hype and hyperbole around new fields of research when they arise.

Marie Kondo Meets Killer Thoughts

With all that in mind, what is the truth behind those very startling accounts, described at the beginning of this chapter, of how nocebo effects can kill? If news stories are taken at face value, those inclined to commit homicide might merely induce the expectation of death in their victims to succeed. Such a tactic might prove the perfect murder. After all, prompting noxious nocebo effects requires no weapons and no fingerprints, only manipulation, leaving crime scene investigators with no forensic trail.

While it is easy to mock the idea of lethal nocebo effects, and although anecdotal reports are prone to exaggeration, the association between nocebo effects and death is surely worth further sleuthing. Indeed, it is only fair that we proceed judiciously to avoid nocebo effects being unfairly blamed when they are not the culprit.

For example, writing in the *British Medical Journal* in 2001, David Phillips and colleagues investigated the influence of what they described as the *"Hound of the Baskervilles* effect."[15] Specifically, they wondered whether unpleasant cultural associations with the number 4 might be associated with higher risk of mortality. Among people from Chinese and Japanese cultures, this number is perceived as unlucky, in the way Americans view 13 as unlucky, and is associated with death. Investigating mortality rates and death certificates dated between 1973 and 1998, Phillips and his team found that on the fourth day of the month cardiac deaths were significantly more frequent than on any other day of the month for Chinese and Japanese Americans, but not for white Americans. Phillips and his team named the phenomenon after Charles Baskerville in the Arthur Conan Doyle novel, who suffered a fatal heart attack caused by extreme psychological stress.

Can we classify the Baskervilles effect as synonymous with the nocebo effect? Interestingly, the investigators did not invoke the idea. They also added the caveat that behavioral changes on the fourth day of the month might have resulted in higher numbers of deaths. They do suggest psychological distress may have caused a rise in fatalities. Still, this could lead to false accusations against nocebo effects. If we frame the idea that nocebo effects resulting in death arise as a consequence of engaging perceptual and cognitive processes about death, the case seems categorically different from pain or nausea. This is because it is unclear what an expectancy—or experience—of death might mean here that renders it a self-fulfilling prophecy. Alternatively, though it is perhaps unlikely, we might still salvage the idea of death by nocebo effect by hypothesizing that the cardiac arrest was the result of specific expectancies associated with experiencing a cardiac arrest, which were genuinely self-fulfilling.

Another option is to loosen up our definitions of nocebo effects to include any adverse health outcomes that arise from engaging perceptual and cognitive processes that influence negative expectancies, which in turn cause negative health outcomes. But if we opt for this, the concept may also become too inclusive and risk redundancy. For now, using Occam's razor, we might suggest that more prosaic explanations are in play. This seems to be what Phillips and co-authors proposed—namely, that the increase in fatalities may simply have been caused by increased psychological distress that day without any outcome-specific expectancies being elicited. This also seems to be the view proposed by Esther Sternberg, M.D., who, writing in the *American Journal of Public Health* in 2002, revisited the idea of "voodoo death."[16] She argued that acute fight-or-flight responses may have induced a cascade of physiological effects. According to Sternberg, an overwhelming release of adrenaline and stress hormones triggered by the brain's hypothalamic stress center could cause cardiac arrhythmias or even vascular collapse, and in rare circumstances even death. So, while the effects were psychosomatic, the suggestion is that not everything psychosomatic constitutes a nocebo effect. As in the Baskervilles effect, in the case of "voodoo death" it may be doubtful that particular expectancies were involved, as opposed to profoundly scary events culminating in extreme physiological stress causing cardiac arrest.

As this case study shows, investigating cold cases in nocebo research is important. And as we have seen, not everything may be justifiably labeled a "nocebo effect." As we continue to explore the nocebo effect, we must emphasize the value of slower, more cautious reflection. In so doing, we can begin to demystify the weird and rather worrying world of nocebo effects.

CHAPTER 5

THE BIOLOGY OF NOCEBO EFFECTS

Luana Colloca, Maxie Blasini,
and Giordana Segneri

A few months ago, I (Colloca) was asked by a reporter to comment on the role of the nocebo phenomenon in Havana Syndrome. The reporter was referring to a set of symptoms experienced mostly by government officials and military personnel that first occurred at the U.S. embassy in Havana.

"Is this a nocebo effect?" the reporter asked. I explained that I had never heard about the disease but wanted to learn about it. I did some quick research, and the syndrome reminded me of other mass psychogenic illnesses (see Chapter 12), whereby people in a group may feel sick as a result of thinking that they were exposed to something dangerous—even though there is no real noxa, or harmful agent.

Nocebo effects are adverse outcomes due to negative expecta-tions.[1] The clearest example of nocebo effects come from placebo treatment in clinical trials. Up to 19 percent of adults and 26 per-cent of older adults report adverse effects when they are given pla-cebos in clinical trials. A quarter of those given a placebo in clinical trials discontinue their participation because of adverse effects. This discontinuation can negatively impact clinical trial enrollment and the ability to retain participants in clinical trials.

In early research, such nocebo responses were regarded as an inconvenient phenomenon that made it hard to test the actual biological activity of medications. However, as research has advanced over the past few years, we have learned that nocebo effects are a common phenomenon in the context of ordinary healthcare as well as in medical research, and in a wide variety of other situations as well. We are now beginning to understand some of the mechanisms—psychological and biological—that give rise to nocebo effects.

Studies in both laboratory and clinical settings, some of which are described in other chapters, document the important role of information and expectations in generating nocebo effects. For example, asthmatic patients who were given a medication called a bronchoconstrictor, which narrows certain airways in the lungs, but who were told that the treatment they received was a bronchodilator (a medication that widens those airways) showed a *widening* of the airways. The opposite is also true: patients with asthma showed a *narrowing* of the airways when the bronchodilator they were given was described to them as a bronchoconstrictor.[2] Along these lines, another paradoxical nocebo response applies to muscle responses. Participants who were told that they had been given a muscle *stimulant* (a medication that increases muscle tone) experienced muscle *tension* even though in reality they had received a muscle *relaxant* (a medication that decreases muscle tone).[3]

Nocebo effects can also affect Parkinson's disease, a condition that causes, among other symptoms, bradykinesia, an extreme slowness of reflexes and movements. Often when medications do not work to reduce these symptoms, Parkinson's patients undergo a neurosurgical procedure called deep brain stimulation involving the placement of electrodes connected to a neurostimulator, which can be turned on and off to deliver electrical impulses. Parkinson's patients in one study were misleadingly told that a deep brain stimulator sending stimulation to a region of the brain called the subthalamic area was turned *off*, but it was actually *on*.[4] Patients told this displayed slowed reflexes/movements, as though the stimulation really had been off.[5]

In the hospital, relieving pain after surgery is critical. In a landmark study, pain treatments were delivered into the bloodstream through an automatic pump, but the patient was unaware of the timing of the infusion. Patients underwent thoracotomy, a surgical procedure, in order to remove lung cancer. In the post-operative period, levels of pain and anxiety peak. Pain is controlled with opioids and non-opioid painkillers. When morphine, an opioid, was interrupted openly (that is, patients were told about the interruption), pain increased substantially. On the contrary, when the interruption of morphine was undisclosed (hidden), the level of clinical pain remained consistently low, as if the opioid had continued being pumped into the bloodstream.[6]

A revolutionary discovery in nocebo mechanisms came with the advent of brain imaging techniques that can depict changes in the brain associated with nocebo effects and shed light on their neural signature. Using the open-hidden procedure described above,[7] a pioneering study indicated that the effects of a strong narcotic such as remifentanil can be completely blocked by the suggestion that the infusion of the drug has been stopped. In one study, remifentanil was continuously infused in the participants' veins, but the participants were told that the drug was discontinued.[8] As expected, participants experienced increased pain (hyperalgesia) after being told the drug had been discontinued. Brain activity was measured with functional magnetic resonance imaging (fMRI). When participants experienced nocebo hyperalgesia, brain activity increased in a part of the brain called the hippocampus, which is involved in learning and memory.[9]

Nocebo effects also depend on the order in which treatments are delivered.[10] Luana Colloca and Fabrizio Benedetti conducted a study in which participants were assigned to one of two groups. Group 1 received a treatment presented as effective, and Group 2 received the same treatment, not presented as effective or ineffective but taken after an ineffective one. The groups differed in the degree of pain reduction (49.3 percent versus 9.7 percent, respectively).[11] Similarly, Simon Kessner and colleagues found that starting a new medication after an unsuccessful medication created nocebo pain increases. The brain processes therapeutic failure with an activation of the posterior insular cortices, areas of the brain related to feeling pain.[12]

Interestingly, the *price* of a medication described as inducing pain is also associated with nocebo effects and brain activation. Alexandra Tinnermann and colleagues showed that marketing a cream (in reality a sham cream) as an expensive one elicited higher nocebo hyperalgesia than a control cream that was marked as less expensive—that is, the expensive medication increased pain. This effect was mirrored by an increase of activity in brain areas that are hubs for the overall experience of pain, suggesting that nocebo effects have a critical role in processes that signal underlying pain sensation.[13]

Nocebo effects aggravate not only pain but also other symptoms, such as itchiness[14] and shortness of breath.[15] Itchiness can be increased by negative expectation, and this worsening is paralleled by more communication between the insula and the periaqueductal gray—two regions of the brain involved in altering the sensation of pain.[16]

At the molecular level, nocebo effects have been linked to the release of a hormone called cholecystokinin (CCK). CCK acts on the brain to increase anxiety. Cholecystokinin also plays a role in temperature regulation. CCK increases during times of heightened anxiety and appears to have a role in nocebo responses.[17] In an early study that explored the effect of suggestions of hyperalgesia, the researchers measured two hormones that rise during stress, adrenocorticotropic hormone and cortisol. The suggestions of pain increased not just the pain itself but also adrenocorticotropic hormone and cortisol. Interestingly, when participants were given a drug called proglumide, which blocks the effects of CCK, pain was also blocked. This result indicates that CCK is a critical component of the nocebo effect.[18] In general, this research points to a relationship between nocebo effects and how anxiety and stress are regulated.

Nocebo effects resulting from patient-clinician interactions may peak in marginalized communities. Janelle Letzen and colleagues looked at non-Hispanic white and non-Hispanic Black participants who were given a placebo and told that the substance would increase pain sensation, that it would decrease pain sensation, or that it would leave the pain unchanged. Non-Hispanic Black participants had lower or no placebo response and a higher pain rating.[19] In terms of biological sex, there is little consensus,[20] with some research suggesting that women are more likely to experience placebo effects,[21] while other studies observed that men are more prone to experience nocebo effects as a result of verbal suggestions.[22]

Mechanistic research on nocebo effects—that is, research on how nocebo effects are produced in the body—has tangible clinical implications. Nocebo effects are the result of neurobiological mechanisms and a cascade of molecules released in the brain. When a clinician communicates with a patient in ways that convey an expectation of negative outcomes, this can induce unwanted, undesirable, and/or unintended nocebo effects. Repeated associations between cues and negative experiences affect the neurobiology of nocebo in a way that makes the brain more susceptible to a modification of symptoms. While there are many factors that influence neurobiological processes that exist outside of an individual's control, understanding why and how these effects are generated can help to bring agency back to the individual to navigate nocebo effects.

CHAPTER 6

HOW THE MIND CREATES NOCEBO EFFECTS

John M. Kelley

There is nothing either good or bad, but thinking makes it so.
—*Hamlet*, Act II, Scene 2

In the Shakespeare quote that starts this chapter, Hamlet suggests that none of our experiences are intrinsically good or bad. Instead, the thoughts and attitudes we have regarding our experiences determine whether we *perceive* them to be positive or negative. This chapter, and indeed this entire book, is concerned with this phenomenon, especially as it applies to the nocebo effect.

Hamlet's musing presents a radical idea. We typically think that our perception of something is an accurate reflection of reality, and in most cases it is. But there are also many other cases in which our perception diverges from the reality we are trying to perceive. One example comes from a phenomenon psychologists call "motivated reasoning." In a classic study of an Ivy League football game between Dartmouth and Princeton, Albert Hastorf and Hadley Cantril showed that, depending on which team someone is rooting for, a particular play might be perceived by one set of fans as an egregious foul and by fans on the opposing side as simply incidental contact.[1] If you've ever, say, been in the presence of both New Yorkers and Bostonians as the Yankees play the Red Sox, you'll understand this intuitively. When we are motivated by our team allegiance to see a particular pitch as a strike, we are more likely to do so than when we are motivated by our team allegiance to see it as a ball.

A second example of the divergence between perception and reality comes from visual illusions. In the famous Müller-Lyer illusion,[2] shown in the left panel of Figure 1, below, our perception is that the horizontal line on the top is shorter than the one on the bottom, but in fact they are exactly the same length (if you are unconvinced, use a ruler to check). Similarly, in the Ebbinghaus illusion,[3] shown in the right panel of Figure 1, the gray circle within the small black circles on the left clearly seems larger than the gray circle surrounded by the larger black circles on the right. But in fact, both gray circles are exactly the same size (again, if you are unconvinced, use a ruler to check). Interestingly, the Ebbinghaus illusion also helps explain why we perceive the full moon as much larger when it is close to the horizon and as much smaller when it is high in the sky. In each of these visual illusions, our subjective perceptions are in conflict with objective reality. Sometimes what we perceive about the world around us is not the same as what is actually there.

Figure 1: The Müller-Lyer Illusion (left) and the Ebbinghaus Illusion (right)

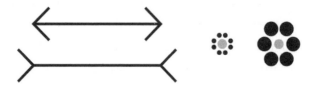

By way of introduction to these ideas as they pertain to medicine, imagine the following common healthcare scenario: At your annual routine physical, your doctor takes your blood pressure and says, "Your pressure is 162 over 96, which is pretty high. I think we should consider putting you on blood pressure medication." She then recommends lisinopril, but she warns you that in addition to its beneficial effect on blood pressure, the drug can also have side effects. She lists the following potential side effects: dizziness, dry cough, headaches, nausea, vomiting, diarrhea, itching, skin rash, and blurry vision. Although your doctor reassures you that these side effects occur relatively infrequently and often diminish or go away over time, you feel a little worried about taking a medicine that can cause so many possible side effects. Your doctor says that the benefits of the drug (i.e., lower blood pressure and a reduction in the likelihood that you will suffer a heart attack or stroke) outweigh the risk of experiencing side effects, which, unlike a heart attack or stroke, are very unlikely to be fatal. After some back-and-forth discussion with your doctor, you decide to take the medication.

If you are like most people, this encounter with your doctor will make you a bit anxious. You are also likely to pay closer attention to your body to determine whether you might be experiencing any of the side effects the doctor mentioned. And if in the weeks following your physical, you do experience a headache or a rash or develop a cough, it's very likely that you will attribute these symptoms to the lisinopril that your doctor prescribed. It's possible that you will even call your doctor and ask about switching medications or perhaps stopping the medication altogether.

All this is reasonable. But what about the possibility that you would have experienced a headache, a rash, or a cough even if you had not been taking the medicine? Maybe your headache is due to stress at work. Maybe your rash is caused by an allergic reaction to the ingredients in a new detergent you're using. And maybe your cough is due to seasonal allergies. Indeed, these sorts of symptoms are commonly experienced by most people, and therefore it's possible that you are not experiencing any side effects at all, but instead you have incorrectly concluded that the drug caused these symptoms, when in fact, it did not. This is symptom misattribution, which is also mentioned in a few earlier chapters. The consequences can be serious and in rare cases even life-threatening. If you needlessly switch medications, it's possible that you will be taking a less effective drug. Or maybe you will even forgo any medication at all. And if you stop taking the drug, very serious consequences could ensue—in the case of high blood pressure, these could include a stroke or a heart attack.

This chapter will focus on two psychological mechanisms for the nocebo effect, *symptom amplification* and *symptom misattribution*.[4] Symptom misattribution, as described above, occurs when a patient experiences symptoms that they *think* were caused by a medical treatment. But in fact, the patient would have experienced the symptoms anyway, even without any treatment. How could a patient make a misattribution like this?

During our daily lives, we all occasionally experience common symptoms such as headaches, fatigue, or heartburn. And oftentimes we are not quite sure what caused those symptoms. However, if we have recently begun a medical treatment, it would be easy to (mistakenly) attribute those symptoms to the treatment.

Symptom amplification occurs when a patient has side effects that may indeed be caused by the medication, but the patient experiences the side effects as more severe or more distressing because they are focusing so intently on their negative experience. At first this may seem difficult to believe—isn't the pain or discomfort an objective consequence of the treatment? But an example will illustrate that this sort of phenomenon is common.

Think of an instance in your life when you experienced a painful symptom such as a strained back, a twisted knee, or a bruised elbow. Wasn't your pain much more tolerable during the day as compared to when you were trying to go to sleep at night? And wasn't the pain less intense when you were having an interesting conversation with a friend or loved one, as compared to when you were spending time alone? Of course, the difference is that when you are sitting alone during the day or trying to get to sleep at night, there are many fewer distractions and you can't help but focus more on your symptoms. You might think: "Is this ever going to get better? Why does it hurt so much? What can I do to make the pain go away?" The net result is symptom amplification.

It's important to note that the nocebo effect is not caused by a person *imagining* that they have symptoms or making symptoms up. Instead, the nocebo effect in this context occurs when a person who is already experiencing symptoms either erroneously attributes those symptoms to the treatment (symptom misattribution) or experiences their symptoms as being more severe than they otherwise would because they are paying closer attention to their body (symptom amplification).

It's also important to recognize that we are all susceptible to these effects, and therefore it is not a sign of being gullible or naive if one experiences symptom amplification and symptom misattribution. In the opening section of this chapter, I tried to make this point by showing that for all of us, our perception of reality does not always line up with reality itself. Recall the examples of visual illusions and diverging views of football plays depending on what team we are rooting for. These phenomena even affect medical personnel. As they learn about the various diseases and disorders of the body, many medical students worry that they might be developing some of these conditions. This occurs so frequently that it has been dubbed "medical students' disease." Given all this, there should be no stigma and no shame for anyone who discovers that they may be experiencing symptom amplification or symptom misattribution. As this chapter will show, knowing that one might be experiencing symptom amplification or symptom misattribution provides an opportunity to reframe side effects of treatment in a way that is beneficial to the patient.

Symptom amplification and misattribution are causally related to other constructs that have been discussed in this book. Figure 2 is a model for the causal chain that leads patients to experience symptom amplification and symptom misattribution, which then lead to a nocebo effect. The causal chain begins when information regarding the potential side effects of the treatment is provided to the patient. The information could be provided by the patient's doctor or nurse, or by their pharmacist (e.g., "This medication sometimes has side effects, including headaches, fatigue, and dry mouth"). But it could also come from friends or acquaintances (e.g., "My side effects from that medicine were so severe that I had to stop taking it!") or from newspaper or television ads (e.g., "Side effects may include nausea, fever, and dizziness"). The patient could also seek out information on side effects on their own by searching the internet or by reading the drug information leaflet that accompanies the medication.

Figure 2: How Symptom Amplification and Symptom Misattribution Work

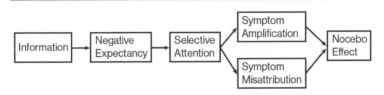

Once the patient has been exposed to information about the possible negative side effects of the medication, they typically form a *negative expectancy*, which simply means that they now expect they might experience some of the negative side effects they have heard about. As a result of this negative expectancy, the patient is likely to pay close attention to whether they have experienced any side effects. This increased focus on symptoms is called *selective attention*. Finally, selective attention to potential side effects is likely to have two effects. First, by paying closer attention and being vigilant for potential side effects, we tend to experience those symptoms more strongly. This is symptom amplification. As an example, when you are exercising, compare the difference in how much muscle pain you feel when you are distracted by watching your favorite TV show versus how much more pain you typically experience if there are no distractions whatsoever. The exertion you are putting into the exercise might be exactly the same (and so the pain "should" be the same), but the distraction provided by the TV show is likely to reduce the pain you feel, and the lack of distraction when there is no

TV will make you pay more attention to the pain and feel it more intensely.

The second effect associated with selective attention is that if you experience a symptom that you have been previously told might be a side effect of treatment, you are very likely to attribute it to the treatment rather than to some other cause. This is symptom misattribution. As I noted at the start of this chapter, nonspecific symptoms such as headaches, muscle pain, and fatigue occur frequently in the general population.[5] If a patient is getting a medical treatment and has received information that headaches are one of the possible side effects, and then if they do indeed experience a headache, they are very likely to attribute it to the treatment, even though it is possible that the headache might have occurred anyway—for example, as a response to becoming dehydrated, or after a long and stressful day. The net result of both symptom amplification and symptom misattribution is a *nocebo effect*.

SIDE EFFECTS OF STATINS

Statins are a class of cholesterol-lowering drugs that are very commonly prescribed by physicians for patients who have high cholesterol (primary prevention) or who have previously experienced a cardiovascular event (secondary prevention). There is considerable evidence for the safety and efficacy of statins.[6] Statins effectively reduce low-density lipoprotein (LDL) cholesterol—the so-called bad cholesterol. There is strong evidence that high levels of LDL cholesterol play an important role in the development of cardiovascular disease.[7] By prescribing a statin, the doctor hopes to decrease LDL cholesterol and reduce the patient's chances of experiencing a heart attack or stroke. Although statins are very effective at reducing LDL cholesterol, many patients stop taking them due to side effects such as muscle aches or joint pain. The question is whether some of these patients would have experienced such "side effects" even had they never taken a statin. In other words, could the nocebo effect explain why many patients stop taking statins?

Fortunately, we have some high-quality clinical data that bear on this question. Judith Finegold and her colleagues at Imperial College London and the London School of Hygiene and Tropical Medicine recently conducted a systematic review that analyzed data from twenty-nine clinical trials in which 83,880 patients were randomly assigned to receive either a statin or a placebo, in double-blind fashion (meaning that neither the patient nor the physician knew whether the tablets given to the patient were statins or placebos).[8] The overall conclusion of the study was: "Only a small minority of symptoms reported on statins are genuinely due to the statins: almost all would occur just as frequently on placebo." For example, symptoms such as nausea, muscle aches, fatigue, diarrhea, and constipation were no more prevalent in the statin group than in the placebo group.

Although this study provides strong evidence that many side effects of statins are actually nocebo effects, it cannot be used by an individual patient to determine whether they have experienced a nocebo effect. It certainly tells individual patients and physicians to be cautious about prematurely stopping statins due to a new symptom such as joint pain that might not be caused by the statin but might instead have been experienced by the patient even if they were not on a statin. To the degree that doctors are aware of these findings, they could use them to reassure their patients that there is a good chance that the symptoms they are experiencing might actually have occurred even without taking a statin. But how might any individual patient determine for themselves whether the symptoms they are experiencing are actually a side effect of the statins they are taking, or whether they might instead be due to symptom misattribution?

Frances Wood and her colleagues at Imperial College London, King's College London, and the University of Sheffield in England recently published an important study in the *New England Journal of Medicine* that focused on the experiences of individual patients and points to a way to leverage these insights about statins and symptom misattribution to benefit individual patients.[9] Sixty patients who had previously discontinued a statin because of side effects were enrolled in the study. The experimenters asked patients to participate in the study for one year and gave them twelve bottles for treatment. Four of the bottles contained a statin (pills with 20 mg of atorvastatin), four contained a placebo, and four were empty, meaning that the patient did not take anything (a no-treatment control). Neither the experimenters nor the patients knew whether a particular bottle of pills contained atorvastatin or a placebo. Each bottle was to be used for a one-month period, with the order of the bottles randomized for each patient. Using a smartphone app, patients were asked to rate the severity of their symptoms every day on a scale that ranged from 0 (no symptoms) to 100 (worst imaginable symptoms). The average symptom severity scores for patients in each condition are shown in Figure 3.

Figure 3: Average Symptom Severity by Treatment

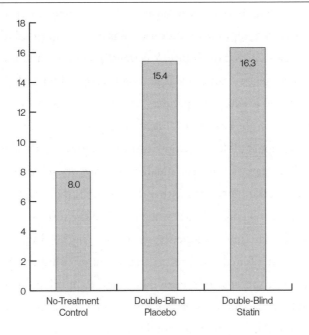

The figure illustrates several important points. The first bar on the left, showing the symptom severity for the no-treatment control, indicates that even in the absence of any treatment at all, many patients often experience symptoms that they might have interpreted as side effects if they were being treated. Second, the fact that the symptom severity scores reported for the placebo were virtually identical to the scores for the statin indicates that the statin did not produce any discernible negative side effects. In fact, taking a placebo resulted in an average symptom severity score that was 94 percent as large as the average score for the statin. This means that 94 percent of the time, a side effect experienced when taking a statin would also have occurred when taking a placebo.

Finally, the fact that the symptom severity scores for the placebo were roughly twice as large as the no-treatment control scores indicates that symptom amplification was occurring. Recall that all patients participated in all three treatment conditions and the order of the treatment conditions was randomly assigned for each patient. Therefore, on average, the patients' symptom severity scores should be the same in the two conditions in which they were not receiving any treatment at all (i.e., the no-treatment control and the placebo). The only explanation for the much higher severity scores when patients were taking placebos is that they thought they might be taking a statin, and consequently when they had the sorts of symptoms that we all sometimes experience, such as fatigue, headache, or joint pain, they attributed them to the statin (symptom misattribution). Furthermore, because of selective attention to possible side effects, they likely experienced the symptoms as more severe than they otherwise would have (symptom amplification).

This study had one other important finding. Six months after the trial ended, 57 percent of the patients had either successfully restarted statins (50 percent) or were planning to do so (7 percent). It's important to remember that all the patients in the trial had previously stopped taking a statin due to intolerable side effects, and yet this intervention helped nearly 60 percent of the patients to restart a statin.

Although this clinical trial was fairly complex, it would be interesting to explore whether the trial's methods could be modified for use in routine clinical practice. In particular, if a patient experienced side effects from a statin medication, the clinician could discuss with the patient the possibility that these symptoms might be due to the nocebo effect. And if the patient was willing, the physician could then institute a mini clinical trial, providing the patient with a blinded statin for some months and a blinded placebo for others, in a randomized order, and having the patient monitor the severity of any symptoms. In this way, some patients might find that the symptoms that they were experiencing on statins were mostly nocebo effects, and more patients would be willing to continue on statins, which would reduce the risk of strokes and heart attacks.

SIDE EFFECTS OF HORMONE REPLACEMENT THERAPY

The thyroid gland produces a hormone called thyroxine, which controls metabolism (the processes through which the body converts food into energy). People with underactive thyroid glands or those who have had their thyroid glands surgically removed don't produce enough thyroxine, and as a result, their metabolism slows down. A slower metabolism causes people to experience symptoms such as weight gain, fatigue, and muscle weakness. Thyroid hormone replacement therapy uses a synthetic (i.e., laboratory-made) version of thyroxine to replace the missing thyroid hormone and alleviate the symptoms.

In 2007, the manufacturer of the most commonly prescribed thyroid medicine in New Zealand changed the formulation of the tablets. There was no change to the active ingredient, but there were changes to the inactive ingredients. In addition, the color of the tablets was changed from yellow to white, and the label was changed from "thyroxine" (the name of the naturally occurring hormone) to "levothyroxine" (the name of the synthetic version).

The labeling change was done to be more accurate; even before the labeling change, the pills had always contained levothyroxine, the laboratory-made version of the hormone.

Remember, the active ingredient had not changed at all. The only changes were cosmetic (i.e., changes in the pill's color, its label, and its inactive ingredients). Nevertheless, there was a spike in reports of side effects from the medication, including symptoms such as headache, nausea, blurry vision, and memory difficulties. Could this increase in reported side effects be a nocebo effect?

Kate Faasse and her colleagues attempted to answer this question by conducting a study that looked at the impact of TV news programs that focused on how often patients reported side effects for thyroid hormone replacement therapy.[10] In New Zealand, the Centre for Adverse Reactions Monitoring collects nationwide data on medication side effects. The study's authors gathered side effects data in the one-month period before, and the one-month period after, a TV news broadcast was aired that reported that patients were experiencing side effects of hormone replacement medication. The researchers were able to collect data for three separate TV news reports that aired between June and September 2008.

The main results are shown in Figure 4. The height of the bars indicates the median number of side effects per day that were reported by patients over a one-month period. White bars are for the one-month period before the TV news reports were aired, and gray bars are for the one-month period after each TV news report was aired. If the side effects were solely due to the medication, then the TV news reports should not have had any effect. But as you can see in the figure, they had a dramatic effect.

Figure 4: Median Number of Side Effects Before and After TV News Reports

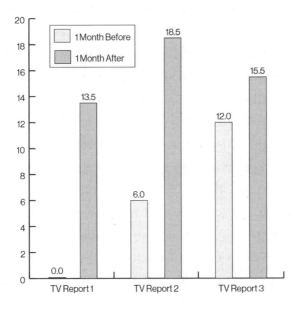

In the one-month period before the first TV news report was aired, the median number of side effects reported per day was zero. This doesn't mean that no symptoms at all were reported. Instead it means that on more than half the days, there were zero reports of side effects. In the one-month period after the first TV news report, the median number of side effects jumped to 13.5. You can see that the same pattern occurred for all three TV reports. In each case, there were many more reports of side effects after a TV news report was broadcast as compared to before. It's also interesting to note that after a TV news report was aired, the median number of symptoms eventually declined after a month or so had passed. It's as though the nocebo effect associated with viewing the TV news reports was gradually wearing off. Importantly, although it is not shown in the figure, the researchers also reported that three months after the last TV report was aired, the median number of symptoms reported per day had dropped back to zero.

These results are persuasive evidence that TV news programs can have a profound impact on patients' experience of side effects. Were patients imagining or making up these side effects? I don't think so. One explanation is symptom misattribution. In other words, it's highly likely that these were symptoms that the patients would have experienced anyway, but because of the TV news reports they had seen, they attributed their symptoms to the thyroid medication. A second explanation is symptom amplification. In other words, patients' experience of preexisting symptoms became more extreme after viewing a TV news programs that focused their attention on possible side effects. Kate MacKrill will explain more about the nocebo effect in the media in Chapter 11.

CHANGING MINDSETS ABOUT SIDE EFFECTS

When a patient experiences unpleasant side effects, they are more likely to stop taking their medication. A promising strategy for dealing with this problem involves changing the mindset that the patient has about side effects. One possible mindset about side effects is that they signal that harm is being done to the body. But an alternative mindset is that side effects, though certainly unpleasant, might actually signal that the medication is working. Does it make a difference which mindset the patient adopts?

To answer this question, Lauren Howe and her colleagues conducted a randomized clinical trial in fifty children and adolescents who were undergoing treatment to reduce their peanut allergies.[11] The treatment is called oral immunotherapy. Patients begin by consuming a very low dose of peanuts, and then slowly increase the dose over a period of six months. The goal is to gradually stimulate the immune system to increase tolerance to peanuts. If successful, this treatment reduces the likelihood that the patient will have a life-threatening reaction if they accidentally eat a food that contains peanuts. Although oral immunotherapy treatment may be beneficial in reducing the risk of a severe allergic reaction, many patients experience mild symptoms during treatment such as congestion, itchiness, or a slight rash. Because these symptoms are similar to a full-blown allergic reaction, they can cause anxiety and lead some patients to stop the therapy.

In the trial, the children and adolescents were informed about potential side effects and how to safely manage them, but half of the patients were encouraged to view their side effects as a signal that the treatment was working and that their bodies were becoming stronger and more tolerant to peanuts. This mindset message was reinforced several times over the course of the six-month trial. Otherwise, the two groups were treated identically.

The results indicated that the mindset intervention was successful. As compared to patients who received the standard treatment, patients who received the mindset intervention reported less anxiety about symptoms, had fewer side effects at high doses of the medication, and were less likely to report that the dosing had not gone well. The mindset group was also less likely to skip or reduce a dose compared to the standard treatment group (4 percent vs. 21 percent, respectively). Finally, the mindset group showed a greater increase in peanut-specific antibodies in their blood, suggesting that they had developed greater immunity to peanuts.

Since this study was relatively small (only fifty patients), it should be replicated in a larger trial to confirm its findings. Nevertheless, the strategy of changing patient mindsets appears to reduce symptom amplification (e.g., mindset intervention patients experienced lower anxiety overall, and fewer allergy-related side effects at high doses). As a result, the mindset intervention increased treatment compliance and increased the benefit of treatment. The mindset intervention works by changing patients' attributions about their side effects from a purely negative interpretation to a more positive one (i.e., side effects signal that the treatment is working). Assuming that these findings can be successfully replicated, this sort of mindfulness intervention has the potential to be used in other conditions to help patients make more positive attributions about side effects and reduce symptom amplification.

Symptom amplification and symptom misattribution are two important causal mechanisms that help explain why patients sometimes experience nocebo effects in response to medical treatment. There is now good research evidence that both of these mechanisms are important factors that cause some patients to experience more frequent and more severe side effects. Other chapters of this book will focus on how these mechanisms can be ethically engaged to reduce nocebo effects. Ultimately, the hope is that patients will benefit by being better able to identify whether they are actually having a side effect to the medication, from a minimization of the severity of any side effects that they are experiencing, and from an increase in the chances that they will be able to continue taking a beneficial medication instead of discontinuing the drug due to negative side effects.

PART THREE

WHAT TO DO ABOUT THE NOCEBO EFFECT

CHAPTER 7

THE ETHICS OF NOCEBO EFFECTS

Marco Annoni

Ironically, "words that make us sick" are often delivered by someone with a medical degree. As previous chapters have shown, clinicians' words may influence a series of symptoms through nocebo effects—from pain[1] and irritable bowel syndrome[2] to headache[3] and sexual dysfunction.[4] For instance, warning a patient that the puncture she is about to receive "will hurt" may increase her pain through nocebo effects. Also, as many of the previous chapters have shown, clinicians' words may be self-fulfilling: describing the adverse side effects of a treatment may bring about these very effects via nocebo mechanisms.

For clinicians, the existence of nocebo effects raises intriguing ethical questions, including the implications of nocebo effects for what is called "informed consent." According to medical ethics and the law, clinicians ought to disclose all essential information for the sake of respecting the patient's autonomy. This is what informed consent means. Such information typically includes a description of the treatment's adverse effects. But as you can now see from the other chapters, these descriptions may harm patients through nocebo effects. This creates an ethical dilemma. On the one hand, a truthful disclosure of treatment adverse effects is needed for informed consent. On the other hand, providing such disclosures may harm patients via nocebo effects, hence violating doctors' ethical duty to "first, do no harm." Doctors cannot eat the informed consent cake and have it too, at least not without sometimes risking nocebo effects.

This ethical dilemma is both fascinating and important. Fascinating, because it vindicates what healers have always known: words are able to change patients' symptoms, alone or in combination with physical remedies. Important, because it points to a fundamental tension in our medical paradigm. This tension pits two irreducible ethical duties against each other: the duty to tell the truth, and the duty to avoid or minimize harm to patients. The tension between these competing ethical values occurs in an endless series of other situations. Besides clinicians, every nurse, dentist, psychotherapist, physiotherapist, and other healthcare professional faces the same dilemma anytime she is communicating with patients about what they may expect from a treatment or the future of their healthcare journey. In all such cases, choosing the wrong words may concretely impact patients' lives through nocebo effects. The result may vary in each individual domain, but the total amount of suffering that could be inflicted or prevented is very significant—as clearly attested, for example, by the case of the adverse effects of COVID-19 vaccines caused by nocebo effects, described in Chapter 3.

FROM PATERNALISM TO AUTONOMY

Imagine you are a clinician. You need to prescribe a patient doxazosin, a common medicine to treat hypertension and symptomatic benign prostatic hypertrophy—an enlargement of the prostate that can cause symptoms such as blocked urine flow and other bladder, urinary tract, or kidney problems. Doxazosin can have various side effects, including dizziness, fatigue, sleepiness, and sexual dysfunction. All these possible side effects are caused by its pharmacological properties. Hence, there is a chance that these adverse effects will occur regardless of whether you inform the patient about them. However, as a clinician, you are also aware that some disclosures might influence nocebo effects. By informing the patient about them, you may increase their chance of occurring and/or their magnitude.

What should you tell the patient? Clearly, one simple option would be to omit any information about these adverse effects. In this way, you would effectively prevent nocebo effects from occurring in the clinician's office. Ethically, this decision could be justified on the basis that providing this information will cause harm without doing any good. Throughout the history of medicine, this practice of filtering out the truth for patients' own good has been labeled in different ways, from doctors' "therapeutic privilege" to "paternalistic deception" or simply "paternalism." In general, "paternalism" can be defined as the intentional overriding of a person's preferences for what is believed to be her own good. The fundamental assumption is that doctors know how to restore and promote patients' health and well-being better than patients themselves. Hence, for patients' own good, sometimes paternalistic doctors must decide *in spite of* or *contrary to* patients' expressed preferences.[5] Classic examples of paternalism are when doctors withhold a negative diagnosis or prognosis to avoid traumatic shocks. And, of course, paternalism occurs also when doctors decide not to disclose treatment adverse effects to avoid nocebo effects.

For centuries, paternalism has been one of the hallmarks of a good doctor-patient relationship. Since the time of Hippocrates, medicine has been traditionally based on two ethical principles. The first was the principle of nonmaleficence ("first, do no harm"); the second was the principle of beneficence ("if possible, help"). Accordingly, a "good doctor" was one who was able to help without causing unnecessary harm. Hippocrates famously said doctors must "conceal most things from the patient. . . . Give necessary orders with cheerfulness and serenity . . . revealing nothing of the patient's future and present condition."

This attitude extended also to the ethics of doctor-patient communication. Healers, quacks, and doctors have always been aware that words were one of the most powerful tools at their disposal— especially at a time when only a few remedies were effective.[6] Like other remedies, words modulate patients' symptoms too. They can convey hope and promote relaxation, or induce despair and increase anxiety and distress. They can be used to persuade patients in choosing the right therapeutic path, or to steer them away from unhealthy habits. Therefore, just like physical remedies, clinicians had to dispense words in a careful and calculated way. And if the truth was judged to be potentially harmful and not helpful, then doctors were usually expected to alter or omit it entirely, in deference to the principle "first, do no harm."

This paternalistic attitude toward doctor-patient communication has been remarkably stable throughout the history of medicine and across different cultures and societies. Consider this staggering account by a young oncologist: "During my first year of oncology fellowship in Italy in 1983, a middle-aged businessman was told he had gastritis, when dying of cachexia from end-stage carcinoma; a young, divorced housewife was told she had arthritis while receiving palliative radiation therapy for chemotherapy-resistant metastatic breast cancer; and a college student was told he had drug-induced hepatitis, but he was indeed progressing toward liver failure from widespread hepatic involvement with lymphoma."[7] In each case the patient's family (or at least one family member) was informed of the truth. Yet these patients were all left in the dark about the severity of their conditions on the assumption that knowing such truth would have done more harm than good to them.

What is wrong in thinking this way? Going back to the prior example, one way of answering this question is to say that by intentionally concealing the adverse effects of doxazosin (or a bad prognosis) you would be jeopardizing another important good: respect for patient autonomy. To clarify this point, we need to unpack why respecting personal autonomy is important and how it relates to informed consent. "Autonomy" is a complex concept, but it is usually defined as the capacity to decide and act according to one's own choices, values, and plans, without external interferences. To be an autonomous agent is to be able to act according to your own values without being coerced or deceived by someone else.

In the last seventy years, personal autonomy has been acknowledged as a fundamental ethical principle alongside nonmaleficence and beneficence. This revolution has been prompted by several factors. One was the public uncovering of unethical experiments involving human subjects, like the infamous Tuskegee syphilis study conducted by the U.S. Public Health Service between 1932 and 1972, in which 600 African American men were "enrolled" with the aim of monitoring the natural progression of the disease. Crucially, none of them was truthfully informed about being part of a study: they were told they were simply being treated for "bad blood." All participants were kept in the dark or explicitly deceived about the true purpose of the medical procedures they were receiving. Obviously, no informed consent was obtained. The study ended only when the press revealed that the participants were left untreated despite a medicine (penicillin) being recognized for decades as an effective treatment for syphilis.

A second factor explaining the rise of autonomy in bioethics was the emergence of a series of civil rights movements during the 1960s and 1970s, first in the United States and then in other countries worldwide. These movements sparked a new social, cultural, and political awareness, which led to increased critical scrutiny of the traditional paternalistic model in medicine. Gradually, the idea that the doctor was the only or ultimate authority on important issues involving the patient's body was increasingly perceived as the relic of a bygone age. Accordingly, the practice of withholding or distorting the truth for patients' own good was also called into question. As many ethical guidelines and codes now state, lying, deceiving, or withholding information from patients is generally considered unethical, unless there are special circumstances in which the good of such paternalistic practices clearly outweighs their cons—such as, for example, in the case in which distressing news is temporarily withheld from a patient who is already having a heart attack.

Today, respect for personal autonomy is paramount in both law and medical ethics, and so are doctors' duties of honesty and transparency. At the practical level, in medicine this entails a recognition that autonomous patients have a right to decide for themselves which medical treatments and information they want to receive or refuse—even if such choices seem to be "against their own good." Hence, before a doctor may proceed with an invasive treatment, patients must provide their informed consent. Consent usually culminates in a written or oral statement that serves as a proxy for the patient's autonomy and as a safeguard against abuses. That is also why you sign an informed consent form before receiving particularly risky or invasive medical procedures.

Consent must always be "informed" because one cannot autonomously decide without knowing one's full array of options and all relevant pros and cons. Clearly, if someone is not informed about the risks and benefits of a treatment, then she cannot make an autonomous decision about whether she wants it or not. Informed consent does not require the communication of every possibly relevant piece of information or potential scenario. In fact, having too much information may impede autonomous decision-making just as much as having too little, a phenomenon that psychologists have described as "information overload" or "cognitive overload." Instead, clinicians should disclose only information that is relevant for patients' autonomous choices. If information can conceivably make a difference for a patient's autonomy, then such information should be part of the disclosure for informed consent. In sum, without truthful and adequate information disclosure one cannot make an autonomous choice, and without an autonomous choice one cannot provide a valid informed consent.

In our example, being oblivious to the side effect of doxazosin may conceivably impact a patient's autonomous choices in different ways. (Recall that all the known side effects of doxazosin may also occur for reasons other than nocebo effects.) For instance, an enhanced risk of fatigue and dizziness may be incompatible with a plan to run a marathon for which the patient has been training so hard in the past months. Also, the fact that doxazosin may induce sexual dysfunction may for some represent critical information in deciding whether to take the treatment. If patients are informed about these possible adverse effects, they might have the opportunity to ask for a different medicine or to postpone treatment. By contrast, if they are left in the dark, they would not be able to make an autonomous choice. In such cases, intentionally concealing information about these side effects would disrespect the patient's autonomy and right to informed consent.

Possible replies to these arguments prioritizing the respect of autonomy are that not every patient is autonomous, or that even autonomous patients may choose to delegate some choices to their doctors. Consider the following real case of a patient we call GC:

> GC is an 89-year-old female nursing home resident with carcinoma of the breast. . . . GC believes her cancer has spread to her bones despite evidence of the contrary. During the admission process, the hospice nurse noted that GC was taking "Cebocap" for pain, which was written by her primary care provider. The nurse was unfamiliar with this medication and looking it up found that it contains "no active pharmaceuticals"—that is, it is a placebo. The patient states, "I can't live without my pain medication," stating that it is quite efficacious for her bone pain. In the hall, the patient's daughters tell the nurse that they know their mother is taking a placebo and do not want it changed. Nor do they want their mother told.[8]

Should the hospice nurse tell the patient that she is taking a placebo? On the one hand, she knows that the patient and her caregivers are fully satisfied with her current regime; on the other hand, she fears that the patient's autonomy is threatened by the administration of the deceptive and inert pill. This dilemma is further complicated by recent discoveries on nocebo effects suggesting that there is a chance for this patient to experience real pain if the doctor withdraws the placebo, and this would require the doctor to prescribe her real analgesics with all their real side effects.

Studies have also shown that attitudes toward truth-telling may vary considerably based on cultural and individual preferences, thus adding another layer of complexity to the ethical dilemmas involving truth-telling in clinical contexts.[9] In general, it is also possible to be fully autonomous and yet prefer to remain unaware of a treatment's potential adverse effects, at least in part because knowing about them may cause unwanted nocebo harm.

With these counterarguments in mind, let us now return to our previous example. It seems that we have only two options regarding the disclosure of doxazosin side effects. One is to intentionally omit all information about them to prevent the nocebo effect. If these side effects are important for the patient's life plans, then omitting such information would fail to respect her autonomy and would be inconsistent with informed consent. The other is to tell the truth and inform the patient about all adverse side effects. This option is consistent with the requirements of informed consent, but it also entails the risk of harm because of the nocebo effect. But are there other options?

According to nocebo scholars and medical ethicists Luana Colloca and Franklin G. Miller, the answer is yes, as doctors may also resort to "authorized concealment." In disclosing the potential side effects of a medicine like doxazosin, a possible strategy is to ask patients in advance if they agree not to receive information about certain types of side effects. Like in a standard disclosure, all serious side effects would still be revealed, as without such information no valid informed consent could be obtained. However, if the patient agrees, all information about mild and transient adverse side effects susceptible to nocebo modulation would be strategically omitted. For example, a clinician could say, "A relatively small proportion of patients who take this medicine experience various side effects that they find bothersome but are not life-threatening or severely impairing. Based on research, we know that patients who are told about these sorts of side effects are more likely to experience them than those who are not told. Do you want me to inform you about these side effects or not?"[10] Authorized concealment allows clinicians to avoid nocebo effects in a way consistent with informed consent and autonomy—even for medicines like doxazosin.

In Chapter 8, psychologists Mette Sieg and Lene Vase of Aarhus University in Denmark will draw on empirical research to weigh whether authorized concealment presents a practical solution to nocebo effects.

NOCEBO EFFECTS FROM THE BEDSIDE TO ONLINE PORTALS

Aside from learning about side effects via doctors' disclosures, patients may discover the adverse effects of treatments in other ways.

One is to be exposed to the media, as will be explained in Chapter 11; another is via the internet. But another, more straightforward way, which arises within healthcare contexts, is by accessing their electronic health records via online platforms. Today, millions of patients have already gained access to their electronic medical records—and many more will follow them in years to come.[11] Electronic medical records may vary in their content depending on the country and healthcare system considered. They usually include scheduled appointments, the results of lab tests, and the list of all prescribed treatments together with their potential adverse effects. In some countries, such as the United States, patients have also access to clinicians' written notes (so-called open notes) as part of their electronic medical records.[12]

Having access to medical records and clinicians' notes has been shown to help patients take more control of their health. More control of their health, in turn, has been correlated with a series of health benefits and may also foster their autonomy.[13] Besides the potential benefits for patients' health and autonomy, however, expanded access to electronic medical records precipitates the question of whether nocebo effects may result from this online information.

In a recent article, philosopher Charlotte Blease has argued that patients' access to their electronic health records and clinicians' notes could potentially elicit nocebo effects in two ways: "first, by facilitating greater understanding about the adverse side effects of their medications and treatments; and second, via negative wording or framing of health information expressed by clinicians in documentation."[14] As for the first aspect, she points to a recent analysis of the largest U.S. survey on open notes: researchers have found that among the more than nineteen thousand patients who were prescribed medications and read at least one note in the previous year, 45 percent reported a better understanding of possible adverse effects of their medications, and 32 percent reported searching for more information about their medications because of reading the notes.[15] These results suggest that a significant portion of patients accessing this documentation online acquire greater knowledge and awareness of the potential adverse effects of their prescriptions. This knowledge may be conducive to many benefits, empowering patients to take control over their health. However, it may also promote adverse side effects because of the nocebo effect, which already occurs in standard clinical settings.

The second route through which electronic medical records and nocebo effects may be related concerns the wording of health information expressed by clinicians in documentation. Studies have shown that after reading their documentation online, some patients may change their mind about the quality of previous therapeutic encounters. For instance, they may start questioning clinicians' competence, whether their condition has been properly diagnosed, and whether they have been stigmatized.[16] It is also well documented that people belonging to minority groups and/or suffering from certain conditions such as obesity are at a higher risk of stigmatization.[17] Electronic medical records may increase the chances of detecting signs of possible stigmatization, as they allow patients to access and compare clinicians' descriptions of their conditions and clinical interactions. In such cases, already vulnerable patients may form negative expectations about future therapeutic encounters. These negative expectations, in turn, may lead to a lower quality of clinical interactions, a factor associated with a greater probability of nocebo effects and lower levels of well-being.[18]

The correlation between expanded access to electronic health records and an increased risk of nocebo effects is yet to be confirmed. However, given the well-established link between these factors in clinical settings, it would be surprising not to find a similar correlation also with respect to online information. Hopefully, future research will help clarify this important issue.

From the standpoint of the ethical dilemma between truthfulness and nonmaleficence, patients' access to electronic medical records and open notes is likely to tilt clinicians' communication further away from paternalism. "Spoken words fly away, written words remain," says the English translation of the classic Latin proverb "Verba volant, scripta manent." In the privacy of a therapeutic encounter, it is relatively easy for clinicians to conceal information. As oral conversations are usually not recorded, clinicians have leeway to decide which information should eventually be concealed or disclosed. For patients, recalling the exact words used to describe the adverse effects of prescribed medications can be difficult and sometimes impossible. Traditionally, this differential access to information has been one of the main grounds allowing for clinicians' "therapeutic privilege," and thus one of the main grounds for medical paternalism.

In contrast, patients' access to electronic medical records and open notes requires clinicians to record this information in an explicit form that will remain accessible 24/7. For patients, it is much easier to double-check, expand on, and compare this information, identifying whether something is missing or is different from how it is reported elsewhere. This is important, for in many clinical settings concealing relevant information without the patient's consent is considered an instance of potential medical malpractice. This creates a strong incentive for clinicians toward more open and transparent disclosures, especially in the case of essential and actionable information such as side effects. Improved access to medical records, thus, may rebalance the traditional power asymmetry between doctors and patients with respect to clinical communication.

In short, traditional clinical encounters are not the only context in which a conflict between truthfulness and nonmaleficence may arise with respect to the disclosure of adverse side effects. Today, the "words that make you sick" may be heard at the clinic as well as read online. At the same time, telling the truth in clinical contexts is no longer considered an exception but the norm. However, in medicine as in life, the same "truth" may be told in many ways, each of which may strike a different balance between truthfulness and nonmaleficence.

ETHICAL RESPONSIBILITIES IN
MANAGING NOCEBO EFFECTS

Every day millions of patients receive a medical prescription or take an experimental treatment as part of a clinical study. These remedies are meant to improve patients' health and well-being but may also cause harm through adverse side effects. In an age in which personal autonomy is a paramount value, clinicians have the duty to disclose these adverse effects so that patients may decide to receive or refuse these treatments. At the same time, as we've discovered, clinicians' disclosures may also harm patients through nocebo effects.

The existence of nocebo effects, therefore, places an important ethical responsibility on health professionals. Living up to this responsibility requires acting on at least three fronts. The first concerns education and professional training. Nocebo effects are ubiquitous in clinical and research settings, and yet information on them is absent from many academic and professional curricula in healthcare. This may lead clinicians and researchers to systematically underestimate the harmful impact that words may have on patients' symptoms. This holds true not only for medical encounters but also in a psychotherapeutic setting (see Chapter 2). Doctors and health professionals should receive adequate training in placebo and nocebo studies with the intent of overcoming the simplistic idea that words are useful only to convey information for the sake of obtaining a valid informed consent.

Patients may profit from better nocebo knowledge too. Being educated about the existence of nocebo effects may aid patients in better contextualizing their symptoms and adjusting their expectations. Preliminary studies suggest that when patients are aware of the existence of expectation-induced nocebo effects, their risk of misattributing unspecific symptoms to treatments may be lower, and this may decrease the number and intensity of such symptoms.[19] Better nocebo education, in sum, may aid in reducing the burden of adverse effects in clinical and research settings.

The second front is empirical research. To date, different techniques have been proposed to reduce nocebo effects caused by information disclosures. Yet more research is needed to compare these alternatives and innovate how informed consent is currently obtained. Designing nocebo-proof disclosures for treatments such as COVID-19 vaccines could reduce the burden of nocebo harm for millions. The same applies to all other disclosures of treatment adverse effects—either oral or written, in person or online. Accordingly, elaborating a list of evidence-based design principles to craft better, nocebo-proof disclosures should become one of the top priorities of nocebo research.

Finally, the third front is ethical awareness. The tension between the duty to tell the truth and the duty not to cause unnecessary harm is intrinsic in all clinical encounters. Better nocebo education and nocebo-proof disclosures may aid in reducing this tension, but they cannot erase it. In many cases, clinicians and health professionals will need to rely on their best clinical judgments to navigate between these conflicting principles. However, this ability requires the cultivation of the appropriate capabilities and skills to balance between respect for autonomy and nonmaleficence without compromising on the most important scope of medicine: to act, always, for patients' good.

CHAPTER 8

HOW CLINICIANS CAN MINIMIZE NOCEBO EFFECTS

Mette Sieg and Lene Vase

In Chapter 7, medical ethicist Marco Annoni explained how clinicians are confronted by a dilemma on a daily basis: how best to inform patients about side effects while avoiding, or at least minimizing, nocebo effects. At an official meeting for experts in the field of placebo and nocebo research in 2018, the consensus was that "information about side effects should be presented in such a way that nocebo effects are minimized" and at the same time efforts should be made to "balanc[e] the need for honesty and transparency with the requirement that harms should not be induced or increased unnecessarily."[1] Simply put, clinicians need to minimize the harmful effect of side effect information in a way that is ethically acceptable. The adage "easier said than done" certainly applies here, but this chapter offers potential solutions to this conundrum by drawing on a variety of empirical research to inform the ethical debate.

How can clinicians minimize nocebo effects? Let us think about what the process of providing side effect information looks like, which for the purpose of this chapter can be split into three components. First, there is the obvious part, where the clinician gives the patient information about potential side effects (we can call this the *information* component). The clinician could target the information component by thinking about what information is given to the patient and how it is presented. Second, side effect information can create negative expectations in the patient, and with this in mind the clinician could aim at optimizing the patient's expectations for the treatment situation (*expectation* component). Last, when the clinician provides side effect information, it does not happen within a neutral space. The context of the situation—for example, the patient's current mood, or the quality of the relationship and interaction between the clinician and the patient—influences how the patient perceives and processes that information (*context* component). All these components influence the nocebo effect and could be targeted by the following nocebo-minimizing strategies:

1. Omission, authorized concealment, and framing of side effect information (strategies targeting the *information* component)
2. Expectation optimization and nocebo education (strategies targeting the *expectation* component)
3. Optimization of the patient-clinician interaction (strategies targeting the *context* component)

Although the information, expectation, and context components in reality overlap and interact, this categorization is used to provide a clear overview when presenting each strategy. Another important thing to keep in mind is that because research on how to minimize nocebo effects in clinical practice is still relatively sparse, it would be premature to offer a fixed set of guidelines to follow. Instead, this chapter presents and evaluates potential strategies based on available evidence of their effectiveness, whether they live up to ethical standards, whether they align with how patients wish to be informed about side effects, and how easy it would be to implement these strategies in daily practice.

INFORMATION STRATEGIES

How can clinicians minimize nocebo effects by considering the information they give to patients? Perhaps the simplest and most straightforward strategy, at least in theory, is to eliminate the harmful thing altogether, as Chapter 7 discussed—that is, to simply omit side effect information. If we do not provide information about side effects, then that information cannot cause nocebo effects and harm the patient.

In fact, this strategy seems to be highly effective at minimizing nocebo effects. A systematic review investigating different strategies for minimizing nocebo effects found that omitting side effect information was the most effective.[2] An example of how effective it can be to omit such information is evident in a classic nocebo study, described in Chapter 1, in which 120 patients who had been prescribed finasteride—a medicine that treats benign prostate enlargement—were split into two groups.[3] Patients in the no-information group reported a smaller proportion of sexual side effects compared to patients who had been informed of these potential side effects during the informed consent process (15 percent vs. 44 percent).

Although omission seems highly effective, its use in real-world patient-clinician situations is obviously problematic. It violates the ethical principle of respect for patient autonomy, which states that patients have a right to be fully informed about a treatment so that they can make an informed decision about whether to agree to the treatment. Nevertheless, regardless of the ethical perspective, as Marco Annoni noted, we need to ask what patients themselves want to know in such a situation. If in fact it turned out that most patients did not really want any information about side effects, then perhaps we could disregard the ethical principle. However, several surveys asking just that show that the majority of patients want to be fully informed about potential side effects.[4] Although some patients say they prefer limited or no side effect information, these belong to the minority. Thus, omitting side effect information, while effective at minimizing nocebo effects, would go against the wishes of the majority of patients.

However, let us for a moment dwell on the minority of patients who prefer to have limited or even no knowledge of potential side effects. Could the clinician then consider omitting such information when interacting with this particular group of patients? Perhaps, if they used the method of authorized concealment,[5] discussed in Chapter 7. To recap: with this strategy, the clinician is open about the fact that the treatment could come with some side effects, but does not mention which ones. Additionally, the list of potential side effects could be written down and put inside a sealed envelope for the patient to keep (and eventually open in case they changed their mind and wanted to know about the specific side effects after all). Yet omission of side effect information, even through authorized concealment, presents another problem: patients should know which symptoms are to be expected but pose no great risk and which symptoms warrant contacting the clinician. One workaround would be for the patient to designate someone (say, their spouse or roommate) with whom they share all their symptoms. Instead of telling the patient about potential side effects, the clinician discloses this information only to the patient's family member or friend.[6]

Although authorized concealment has been widely discussed as a potential strategy for minimizing nocebo effects, there seem to be no investigations into whether it would actually work. On the face of it, this strategy resembles that of omission—information about side effects is being withheld—and we know that omission works. Think back to the finasteride study. However, we need to consider the fact that *knowing* that side effect information is available but not knowing *what it is* may itself have some sort of effect. Perhaps this leaves some patients even more worried and prone to experiencing nocebo side effects because they imagine risks far worse than those being concealed.[7] Furthermore, findings from the psychology of confidentiality have shown that flagging and then concealing information intensifies the desire to uncover it, especially when that information is personally relevant. So, the awareness that side effect information is available but has been concealed may for some patients increase interest in uncovering this information. Once uncovered, this information may cause the nocebo effects that authorized concealment was meant to avoid in the first place.[8]

Let us consider a different strategy. Rather than thinking about *which* information to present, the clinician could focus on *how* information is presented, because it may be possible to present side effect information in a way that does not cause nocebo effects. Such information is usually presented as the proportion of people who experience a given side effect (e.g., "three out of ten people *will* experience nausea"). With positive framing, the same risk information is presented, but instead as the proportion of people who do *not* experience the side effect ("seven out of ten people will *not* experience nausea"). By using positive framing, all information is available to the patient, but the idea, in theory, is that it is less likely to induce negative expectations of experiencing side effects.

So, is this method effective? The short answer: maybe. Although positive framing is an interesting strategy, relatively few studies out there have actually looked into it. A systematic review from 2019 found only four studies on this type of positive framing, of which three found that positive framing was somewhat effective.[9] Although more studies have joined the discussion in the last few years, the picture is still unclear. For example, one recent study presented the risk of nausea for a virtual-reality task.[10] The researchers found that positive framing ("seven out of ten people will *not* experience nausea") worked as predicted and reduced nausea compared to negative framing ("three out of ten people *will* experience nausea"). They even found that positive framing was as effective as omitting side effect information. In another recent study, the risk of headache in relation to sham brain stimulation was presented as "70 percent *likely* to occur" (negative framing) or "30 percent *unlikely* to occur" (positive framing).[11] Here, positive framing was *not* effective at minimizing side effects when side effect occurrence was assessed during the brain stimulation, though reports of side effects were somewhat reduced when assessed *after* the procedure, suggesting that retrospective measures could be more influenced by framing. This should illustrate that findings on positive framing are mixed— sometimes it works well, sometimes it does not, and why this might be the case is still unclear.

Once we get a better understanding of framing, it could be a promising way of minimizing nocebo effects, especially since no information is being withheld and it would be easy to adopt the strategy in clinical practice. We are currently conducting a survey to investigate whether patients find this method acceptable. Yet there is still an ethical perspective to consider: whether, and how, positive framing affects the way people perceive risk.[12] Evidence suggests that risk information is perceived differently depending on how it is presented and framed. For example, one study found that patients perceived a medicine as less risky when side effect information was framed positively versus negatively,[13] although it is uncertain which framing leads to the most accurate risk estimation. From an ethical perspective, positive framing—and the more commonly used negative framing, for that matter—should be considered acceptable only if it does not interfere with the patient's ability to correctly interpret the risks. Therefore, we need more studies investigating the effect of framing on side effect occurrence as well as on risk perception relative to actual risk, in order to consider how framing could be used in clinical practice.

Each of the three strategies reviewed so far—omission, authorized concealment, and positive framing—has pros and cons. While omission seems to be an effective way of minimizing nocebo effects, its implementation in clinical practice is not realistic because it goes against patient autonomy and general patient wishes. Authorized concealment could be a potential alternative for the minority of patients who prefer limited side effect information, but we still lack empirical studies assessing its effectiveness. Last, positive framing is an interesting strategy in which patient autonomy is preserved, but research is mixed as to how well it works. It is also uncertain how framing may influence patients' risk perception.

EXPECTATION STRATEGIES

When the clinician provides side effect information, it may exaggerate the patient's *expectations* of experiencing side effects, which in turn may cause nocebo side effects. A recent study found that 83 percent of participants expected to experience the side effects they had been warned about.[14] Yet people could be overestimating their own likelihood of experiencing side effects that they have been warned about and therefore may have unrealistically negative expectations. This invites questions about whether clinicians could minimize nocebo effects by optimizing patient expectations. Here, we take a look at two potential strategies that target patients' expectations about side effects: expectation optimization and nocebo education. Through conversation, the clinician may discover that the patient's expectations about the course of their condition and/ or preconceptions about an upcoming treatment are unrealistically negative. The clinician can try to optimize the patient's expectations by providing realistic information and talk about the benefits of the treatment. Thus, the goal of expectation optimization is to reduce maladaptive expectations (such as exaggerated expectations of side effects) and enhance adaptive expectations. A systematic review has investigated the effect of expectation optimization on different clinical outcomes such as return to work, anxiety, depression, and illness-related disability.[15] Although not specifically in relation to side effects, the review found that expectation optimization generally improved clinical outcomes, and it could be a promising strategy for minimizing nocebo side effects. However, expectation optimization is relatively time-consuming, as it entails several sessions with a healthcare provider prior to having a procedure or being prescribed a new drug. Consequently, at least in its current form, it is not something that could be easily and widely implemented in clinical practice. However, with more studies and more knowledge about its effectiveness, this approach might be something to consider in certain patient populations who must undergo invasive and expensive treatments, where recovery is prolonged and the burden of side effects can be severe.

So, let us turn our attention to a simpler, less time-consuming expectation strategy: nocebo education, also discussed in Chapter 7. The idea is that when warnings about side effects are presented, patients are also educated about nocebo effects. That is, patients are made aware of the fact that side effect information itself can be the cause of more side effects. The rationale behind this strategy is that patients may be less affected by the side effect information if they are aware of the power of their own expectations. Not much research has looked into the effectiveness of nocebo education. But one study found that participants with chronic headaches experienced fewer side effects from a placebo treatment when they learned about the nocebo effect during the informed consent process.[16] Furthermore, a recent study found that nocebo education reduced the number of side effects reported twelve weeks after starting chemotherapy for gastrointestinal cancer.[17]

As mentioned, in these studies nocebo education seems to work by changing patients' expectations about side effects. Besides that, nocebo education may also minimize nocebo effects in another way, by reducing patients' desire for side effect information—and, as we know by now, less information about side effects means fewer or less problematic nocebo side effects. This "indirect" effect of nocebo education is seen, for example, in a study investigating participants' desire for information related to an antidepressant.[18] In this study, a group of participants presented with a description of nocebo effects desired less information about side effects and were more likely to agree that withholding side effect information could be beneficial, compared to a group of participants who were not presented with information about nocebo effects.

From an ethical point of view, nocebo education is a promising strategy for minimizing nocebo effects, as it allows for the informed consent process to remain intact. In addition, nocebo education is simple and relatively easy to implement in clinical practice. Although this is a promising strategy, very few studies on nocebo education exist, highlighting a need to investigate whether nocebo education is indeed effective at minimizing nocebo side effects.

CONTEXT STRATEGIES

Can clinicians minimize nocebo effects by targeting the context within which the patient receives information about side effects? From the moment they enter the clinic, patients are met with impressions that may influence their psychological state. For example, the waiting room may trigger memories of previous treatment experiences and cause anticipatory anxiety. A patient who is anxious and stressed may be more likely to experience nocebo effects,[19] and a patient's current mood may be important for how sensitive and receptive they are to side effect information. A study looked at the effect of warning versus not warning patients that they might experience a headache from the sham brain stimulation they were about to undergo.[20] But before that, half the participants had watched a happy video designed to put them in a positive mood state, and the other half had watched a neutral video. Of those who had watched the neutral video, the side effect warning increased nocebo headaches compared to no side effect warning. This is another example of how omitting side effect information can minimize nocebo effects. What is most interesting about this study is the results from the participants who watched the positive video. Here, the side effect warning did *not* increase nocebo headaches as it did in participants with neutral mood. That is, making sure that the participants were in a positive mood blocked the negative impact of side effect information.

When meeting and interacting with a patient, the clinician could think about how to improve the patient's psychological experience of the interaction. As there seems to be negligible research on the patient-clinician relationship in relation to nocebo side effects, let us for a moment draw on what we know from placebo research. In one study, the researchers first induced a small allergic reaction on the arm of the participants, followed by the application of a sham cream.[21] Participants were told that the cream would reduce the allergic reaction. When the clinician showed both warmth and competence, the allergic reaction decreased in size compared to when the clinician seemed cold and incompetent. This study reflects a common finding from scientists who study the placebo effect—that a positive interaction and relationship with the patient has positive patient health outcomes.[22] Since it has been suggested that a poor patient-clinician relationship may do more harm than a good relationship does good,[23] it is important to start investigating how the patient-clinician interaction may influence nocebo side effects.

Another thing that could fall within the patient-clinician interaction and influence nocebo effects is the expectations of the *clinician*. This was shown in a study of patients who received a sham drug to relieve their pain following the removal of a wisdom tooth.[24] The clinicians were told that in one of the patient groups, the drug they were administering could be either a pain-*enhancing* drug or a sham drug. For the other group of patients, clinicians were told that the drug could be either a pain-*enhancing* drug, a pain-*reducing* drug, or a sham drug. That is, only in the latter group did clinicians believe that patients had a chance of experiencing pain relief. Corresponding with the *clinicians'* expectations, patients in the latter group experienced greater pain relief even though everyone received a placebo. It seems that patients may notice subtle cues reflecting the clinician's expectations about a treatment, which may influence the patient's own expectations. Relevant to this chapter, it raises the question of whether a clinician's own expectations about a patient's likelihood of experiencing side effects could similarly have an effect on the occurrence of nocebo side effects.

Of the three components highlighted in this chapter, the *context* component is certainly the one that has received the least attention in the nocebo literature. More research on this has been conducted in relation to placebo, so we might be able to make some preliminary assumptions. An ethical advantage of targeting context components compared to some information components is that it does not compromise the patient's right to be informed about side effects. The idea is that while warning the patient about potential side effects, the clinician can modify her own expectations and behavior to create a comfortable, positive environment, putting the patient in the best psychological state to receive side effect information.

WHAT DO WE KNOW AND WHERE DO WE GO FROM HERE?

Clinicians across all healthcare professions—doctors, surgeons, nurses, psychotherapists, dentists, or any other you can think of—may every day in their clinical practice unwillingly and unintentionally be increasing their patients' risk of experiencing side effects. This chapter set out to get closer to answering the question of how clinicians can minimize nocebo effects. And while the focus was solely on nocebo *side* effects—that is, the side effects caused by being informed of potential side effects—let us keep in mind the other types of nocebo effects that might occur in clinical practice. For example, a clinician uses harsh wording to warn that a procedure will be painful, and as a result of these words, the patient experiences more pain than when the warning is presented more gently.[25] A clinician's words can even completely block the effect of a strong painkiller by saying that the administration of the drug has stopped, although in reality the treatment continues.[26] These are other examples of nocebo effects occurring in clinical practice, where clinicians could similarly focus their efforts. Yet—and this goes for nocebo side effects as well—astoundingly little evidence of nocebo-minimizing strategies exists when thinking of how big a difference they could make in the lives of many patients.

However, as Charlotte Blease argued in Chapter 4, nocebo effects are difficult to investigate due to the ethically questionable nature of experiments that aim to induce negative effects. This plays one part in our sparse knowledge of nocebo-minimizing strategies. On top of this, when wanting to minimize nocebo *side* effects, we automatically tap into another ethically sensitive area regarding patients' right to know about both the positive as well as the negative aspects of a treatment option. This partly explains why most (though not all) research on how clinicians can minimize nocebo effects has been carried out in healthy participants and not patient populations. While the existing experimental work is a good and important initial indicator, nocebo-minimizing strategies also need to be tested clinically in real-life patients, who may or may not respond in a similar way to healthy participants.

Nonetheless, there *are* several potential strategies that (once we have collected more data) could be useful for clinicians in their interactions with patients. While we already know that, for example, omitting side effect information is pretty effective, this strategy does not live up to either ethical or patient standards. Instead, learning more about the workings of strategies such as authorized concealment, positive framing, nocebo education, and context optimization could eventually guide us toward ethical, patient-favored, and clinically feasible ways that clinicians can minimize nocebo effects.

CHAPTER 9

PROTECTING YOURSELF FROM NOCEBO EFFECTS

Wayne B. Jonas and Steve Bierman

Most doctors don't realize they may be causing harm with their words, and they would be appalled if they understood this. Nevertheless, it happens frequently in healthcare encounters. You can help to reduce the chances of what is called "doctor-induced nocebo" happening to you.

Let's start with an example of a series of routine patient encounters that illustrate how harm is often caused inadvertently.

MEET CHARLES

Charles is a fifty-two-year-old man with stage III colorectal cancer. First, Charles gets the news from his internist.

> *Internist: Well, Charles, I'm afraid I have some bad news. You have colon cancer, and it is stage III, which means it has started to spread. Best thing we can do is get you to a specialist right away and try to prevent things from getting any worse. I'll be referring you to a great oncologist, so let's be hopeful and try to think positive.*

The word "cancer" is fraught with fear in our society. Just by saying "bad news . . . you have cancer," the doctor is subtly reaffirming the cultural assumptions that a diagnosis of cancer is a death sentence. Cancer is a serious disease, but delivering the diagnosis in this way exacerbates the nocebo-inducing factors already embedded in our culture.

The idea that cancer is always a fatal disease is further reinforced when Charles's oncologist improperly uses statistical information about groups to predict what Charles, an individual, will likely experience.

> *Oncologist: Hi, Charles. I'm glad your doctor got you here so quickly. Your tumor looks like it's aggressive, so we need to start treatments as soon as possible.*
>
> *Charles: Um . . . what treatments?*
>
> *Oncologist: Well, first, surgery. I'll have you see an excellent surgeon tomorrow and we'll schedule the operation as soon as possible. Then, once you're all healed up, we will need to start chemo. As you probably know, this can be kinda tough. But I'll be with you, and we'll try to limit your discomfort and get you through it. Don't worry: before we start, we'll talk over all the complications and how we will try to lessen them.*
>
> *Charles: It's all so sudden and scary, Doc. What are my chances?*
>
> *Oncologist: Honestly, about three out of four people die from your kind of tumor. But that leaves you with a 25 percent chance of survival. And the sooner we start treatment, the better.*

Nocebo effects are often produced by the misinterpretation of probability data—that is, data derived from large groups of people to determine averages and other statistical outcomes. But the oncologist cannot know from group data what Charles, a unique individual, will experience. Misuse of statistical information not only can induce harm but also is an erroneous extrapolation. For example, in this case, the oncologist takes the average five-year survival data for patients with colorectal cancer throughout the country (as derived from national databases) and concretely declares, "That leaves *you* with a 25 percent chance of survival." This is a misinterpretation of probability data and an inaccurate communication of that data, as it assumes the oncologist "knows" that Charles will be "average." The oncologist has no way of knowing where on the probability curve Charles will fall. And yet, by giving specific data as if it applies directly to Charles, rather than presenting it as a population-level generalization, the doctor is predicting Charles's outcome in a way that is erroneous. This is a form of nocebo suggestion.

During the interaction, the oncologist also implies that Charles will likely get sicker over this period: "As you probably know, this can be kinda tough." Then he makes matters worse by adding: "We'll try to limit your discomfort and get you through it." But the word "try" implies an obstruction, and thereby conveys the notion that the oncologist may only have limited success with Charles. This, then, is felt by Charles as something like a curse, albeit unintended, that he will experience a "tough" time and "discomfort." The oncologist has no way of knowing this. Charles may, in fact, be genetically, socially, behaviorally, or intrinsically different from every other patient the doctor has ever seen. Yet Charles, who is now in an extremely vulnerable state, is quite likely to absorb the information this doctor is conveying and be harmed by the way it is delivered.

Finally, with respect to this encounter, the oncologist has named Charles's cancer "your tumor," instead of, say, "the tumor." This wouldn't matter if words didn't matter, but, as you will see, they most certainly do. Therefore, locating the tumor within Charles's self-conception is also potentially nocebo-inducing.

Next, Charles sees the surgeon, and additional deleterious ideas are layered on.

> *Surgeon: Hi, Charles. Well, your doctors are right. You have an aggressive*
> *tumor by all accounts. We should remove it as soon as possible.*
> *Charles: Okay.*
> *Surgeon: So, let me tell you the risks so you can be informed, and then*
> *I'll have you sign a consent.*
> *Charles: Um . . . okay.*
> *Surgeon: Truth is, like all surgeries, there's a risk of bleeding. Of course,*
> *I'll do all I can to try to prevent that. But you could bleed. You could*
> *even lose a lot of blood. And this can lead to transfusions, or, in rare*
> *cases, you could even die. Remember, I have to inform you of these*
> *risks, but they are rare.*
> *Charles: I understand.*
> *Surgeon: Good. Then, after the surgery there is, naturally, pain.*
> *Sometimes severe. But we have strong medicines for that and will try*
> *to keep you comfortable throughout your convalescence.*
> *Charles: And how long will that be?*
> *Surgeon: Well, the surgery is extensive, so sometimes recovery can be quite*
> *long. You might need months or even a full year to really feel and act*
> *like normal again.*

In the spirit of transparency, the surgeon tells Charles that there are extensive risks from his surgery. "You" could have a large amount of bleeding, with the possibilities of needing a transfusion and even bleeding to death. Charles is also told "you" may have severe pain afterward, which will be treated with strong painkillers. Finally, the surgeon tells Charles that "you" will have a prolonged recovery and follow-up period, during which time he will not feel "normal."

All these statements are communications to Charles that may or may not reflect his actual outcome. Yet the data have shown that these communications, as they are currently stated, can influence the likelihood of them occurring. Multiple studies have shown that giving patients information about the side effects of a treatment increases the rate at which patients experience those side effects.[1]

The reality is that "some people" have bleeding, severe pain, and protracted recoveries. Not all people, and perhaps not "you." However, when an authority communicates by using the word "you," it pins the possibility of an adverse event on the patient. "You" could bleed. "You" could hurt. "You" could suffer. "You" could die.

It would be far better, and more accurate, to say, "Some people bleed. Some have pain. Some, rarely, die. We are always here to help. And, for all we know, you will have a perfectly smooth course. Let's see how well you do." (More on this later.)

Finally, after surgery, Charles returns to his oncologist for chemotherapy. Once again, an authority figure gives him information.

Oncologist: Well, Charles, I'm glad you're back and ready to start chemo. The ordeal isn't over yet, but we're getting there. As I said in the

*beginning, chemo can be tough. But I'll be with you through it, and
we'll try to keep the unpleasantness to a minimum.*

Charles: *I'd certainly appreciate that, Doc.*

Oncologist: *So, listen, here's what we'll be dealing with. This chemo can really
put you back on your heels for a while. You'll probably lose your appetite
and suffer nausea and vomiting. We'll treat that with medicines and, if
it's necessary, with IV fluids. You'll also most likely experience hair loss and
profound weakness and lethargy. That, you'll just have to tough out. But in
the end, we are trying to kill this cancer and give you a few more good years.*

Charles: *I know, Doc. Thanks.*

When the oncologist says he will "try to keep the unpleasantness
to a minimum," he is implying not only that there will be unpleasantness but also that there will be some obstruction to his efforts
to minimize it. Still, he'll "try." Further, the "you will" statements
that follow this inadvertent suggestion of "unpleasantness" set up
expectations of nausea, vomiting, hair loss, and weakness. Finally,
as if that's not bad enough, the oncologist unwittingly extinguishes
the hope of a cure by suggesting that, at best, this treatment will buy
Charles "a few more good years."

Charles and patients like him take on a slew of negative suggestions during their interactions with healthcare workers. These
suggestions can be directly harmful, even though the clinicians'
intentions are simply to inform their patients accurately.[2] As our
example of Charles's interactions shows, the various types of communications in which nocebo effects can be produced often occur
through routine doctor-patient encounters. Shortly we will illustrate
not only how these nocebo effects can be avoided and minimized

but also how these same communications can be restructured to enhance healing and reduce adverse effects.

PREVENTING NOCEBO EFFECTS

Educating Your Caregiver

Most clinicians are compassionate people. When they offer a negative suggestion, it is rarely on purpose. Often they simply do not understand the full meaning and impact of their words. After all, clinicians are not taught the nuances of language, nor are they taught the limitations of their knowledge or the impossibility of predicting the future. Instead, most believe that general facts and compassion will suffice when communicating with patients. Sadly, compassion is not enough. In fact, once vested with authority, clinicians need to attend scrupulously to the impact of their communications, lest harm be done.

We can help prevent our clinicians from misspeaking by politely educating them about their statements. For example, one patient who was too shy to speak face-to-face with her specialist timidly handed him a card that read: "Dear Doctor, my present condition has me worried and, I think, particularly vulnerable to any negative suggestions. You have always been kind and well-intentioned toward me. Let me ask you now to please take particular care with your words. They are very powerful, and I only want to hear positive words at this time. Thank you so very much for understanding." Any communication of this sort with your clinician—an email before your visit, a card handed to the intake nurse, and so on—will remind them that their words matter.

However, working under pressure, even the most well-trained clinician will sometimes misspeak. It is inevitable. So, to prevent their unintended comments from doing us harm, we need to inactivate their persuasive influence. Fortunately, our simple understanding of nocebo effects and how they are magnified in the clinical situation makes that possible.

Empowering Yourself

Regardless of your diagnosis, you are still you—a sovereign individual endowed with reason, will, and choice. You are the one who must choose your course of treatment. You are the one who will decide whom to trust and whom not to trust, where to go and where not to go, what to do and what not to do. You are unique, and you are in charge of you. Retain your agency no matter the diagnosis. You are not helpless. And you need only depend on those you choose to depend on.

In this connection, if you have the choice, it may benefit you to choose a medical establishment that is not dehumanizing. Many medical establishments, by virtue of their proportions, reputation, or culture, induce a sense of insignificance and smallness in patients. Other medical establishments, regardless of size and scope of care, feel warm and welcoming to patients.

When you retain your sovereignty and move about in comfortable, respectful surroundings, you are far less vulnerable to the primordial dependency/authority response pattern that drives nocebo effects.

Do Not Vest Too Much Authority in Your Caregivers

Realize that physicians are only experts in rather restricted realms of knowledge: surgery, internal medicine, gynecology, and so on. They are not necessarily experts in other fields of science. Nor are they experts in all the modalities of treatment that lie outside their realms. Most important, they are not experts in *you*. In fact, almost all their expertise derives from their narrow anecdotal experience and from the studies they have read—studies that draw statistical conclusions from the outcomes of groups in which you were not a participant. You may have a unique gene, a distinguishing capability, a different lifestyle, a special support system, a positive mindset, or a bouquet of protective supplements. You may have any number of characteristics and capabilities that distinguish you from the groups your clinician's knowledge is based on. Therefore, it is better to regard your doctors *not* as authorities but rather as consultants, as vendors of advice and counsel. And since your health is your most important project, feel free to consult with as many such vendors as you see fit and are able. When they perform as needed, retain them. When their performance is undesirable, discharge them. You decide. As Dr. Andrew Weil once said, "It is generally not a good idea to retain a doctor you do not feel comfortable with."[3]

In this respect, do not be fooled by their apparent certainty. The practice of medicine is truly an impossible task. The good doctor, one who is doing his or her best in every moment, nonetheless realizes the enormousness of the job. And so, humility is their hallmark. The doctor who is comfortable saying "I don't know" is less likely to harm you with their words than a blind "expert" who pretends to have all the answers. Therefore, value humility in your caregivers.

Erect Some Safety Shields

Even the best clinician will sometimes misspeak. So you need a shield of sorts to prevent their negative suggestions from penetrating.

Here are two such shields: the first deflects the negative comments, the second disrupts the identification that often forms between patient and clinician once the dependency/authority response pattern is activated.

First, remind yourself that you are the expert on who you are, not the doctor. This will blunt the power from whoever is in the process of uttering something untoward. They may be an authority on how a certain condition affects a certain group, but they truly do not know you. And they cannot know your future. (Realize, they don't even know their own tomorrow.) Even if the speaker is a clinician whom you admire, if they are casting negative comments inadvertently, say to yourself as they speak, "You don't know *me*."

Second, bonding and identification with the designated authority often occur spontaneously. These processes may be, and often are, active between you and your doctor, without either of you knowing it. Therefore, at the time when undesirable words are coming at you, break your rapport. Consciously change your behaviors so they do not mirror those of the speaker. If he or she is sitting, then stand. If you are looking at each other, break eye contact. If his or her posture somewhat mimics yours, change your posture. In other words, establish physical dissimilarities that disrupt identification and, thereby, disempower the nocebo suggestions from taking hold.

Defying authority (with an internal mantra) and disrupting identification (by changing your behaviors) are ways to ensure that your clinician's information has less nocebo influence and is delivered solely to your conscious faculties, where it can be weighed on the scales of reason. When this authority pattern is diminished or disallowed by a patient who chooses to retain agency over their healthcare, when identification is disrupted by a patient vigilant to the accidental misspeakings of their caregivers—that is, when the primordial response pattern that drives ideas to actualization is blocked—then nocebo effects are much less likely to occur.

BACK TO CHARLES

Now, let's see how our new understandings can alter the messages Charles receives from and delivers to his caregivers. Aware that their words are imbued with a powerful influence, that ideas can and do affect outcomes, clinicians will speak more carefully and deliberately. Aware that they can retain agency over their own health and direct their own healthcare consultants toward positive outcomes, patients like Charles will be more forthcoming and direct.

Previously:

Internist: Well, Charles, I'm afraid I have some bad news. You have colon cancer, and it is stage III, which means it has started to spread. Best thing we can do is get you to a specialist right away and try to prevent things from getting any worse. I'll be referring you to a great oncologist, so let's be hopeful and try to think positive.

Now:

Internist: Well, Charles, we have a diagnosis. But before I share that with you there is one very important thing I need you to know.

Charles: That's fine, Doctor, but please keep it positive. I feel a little vulnerable right now and really do not want to hear any negative suggestions.

Internist: Of course, and right you are. What I want you to know is that wonders, miracles, and positive outcomes—these things happen literally every day in medicine. And for all I know, Charles, you are the next wonder I will witness.

Charles: *I intend to be.*

Internist: *Unfortunately, we did not get the diagnosis we might have hoped for. It is cancer, and it appears to be stage III, which means it has spread. Fortunately, we have medicines and surgeries that can both stop the spread and, as I said, in many cases work wonders. I'll have you see an excellent surgeon and oncologist, of course, but you should know I will be with you through your entire course.*

Charles: *I appreciate that, Doc. What are my chances?*

Internist: *Charles, we can only truly know that about any individual when we look back. It is true that in general, one person—perhaps very much like you—in every four survives. Of course, there are probably subgroups that do considerably better, and, I suppose, some subgroups that might do worse. Together, we'll do everything we can to make you a survivor. And I will not be at all surprised if one day, we look back on this moment with relief and triumph.*

This is clearly an internist who appreciates the near-hypnotic influence of his communication. His speech is deliberate and prudent— no inadvertent casting of curses. Unfortunately, the oncologist below has not cultivated those same skills. Nevertheless, observe how Charles handles this difficult situation.

Oncologist: *Hi, Charles. I'm glad your doctor got you here so quickly. Your tumor looks like it's aggressive, so we need to start treatments as soon as possible.*

Charles: Well, I'll be interested to hear your thoughts. I'll also be seeking multiple other opinions before I decide what to do.

Also, if you don't mind, it's not "my tumor." It is "the tumor." I know that might seem like splitting hairs, Doctor, but it is a foreign thing, not a part of me, that my immune system and my healing systems must expel.

Oncologist: That's fine. Now, once you're all healed up from surgery, we will need to start chemo. As you probably know, this can be kinda tough. But I'll be with you, and we'll try to limit your discomfort and get you through it.

Charles (who has been thinking throughout this exchange): "You don't know me. You don't know me"): You mean if I have discomfort, don't you? Surely, everyone is different.

Oncologist: Yes, of course. Now, don't worry. Before we start, we'll talk over all the complications and how we will try to lessen them.

Charles (politely standing up and breaking eye contact while the doctor remains seated, thus disrupting any unintended identification): I appreciate that, Doctor, but it's not just potential complications I'd like to learn about, it's also the potential benefits. You'll discuss those, too, won't you, please?

Oncologist: Of course, gladly.

Charles: Wonderful. And as to "trying" to lessen potential complications, I truly appreciate that. Just know that I'll be taking additional measures of my own to be sure it all goes smoothly.

As you can see, this is a changed Charles. No longer has he surrendered agency over his health and subordinated his will to the will of a supposed authority. Instead, he politely retains his sovereignty: informing his caregivers that each of them is but one among many, and that he, Charles, will decide whom to listen to and whose advice to follow. Moreover, Charles shields himself against unintentional negative communications from his caregivers by (1) quietly reciting "You don't know *me*" as the doctor accidentally misspeaks and (2) consciously breaking identification and gently asserting his needs and intentions. This is a Charles whose fate will be determined not by the unintended nocebo effect of an ill-formed communication but rather by warm and reasoned interactions between himself, as agent, and the various providers of his healthcare advice.

Nocebo communications are unfortunate accidents within the healthcare environment. However, by initiating protective measures, you can begin to form new and healthy patterns of interacting with those compassionate, albeit imperfect, caregivers who truly hope and intend to help. Moreover, you will be doing your caregivers (and, consequently, their other patients) a favor—by making them even better healers.

PART FOUR
THE BIGGER PICTURE

CHAPTER 10

NOCEBO, THE ENVIRONMENT, AND PUBLIC HEALTH

Jarry T. Porsius

On Thursday, November 12, 1998, a high school teacher came to work in McMinnville, Tennessee, and noted a "gasoline-like" smell in her classroom. Shortly thereafter she experienced headache, nausea, shortness of breath, and dizziness, and several students in her class soon developed similar symptoms. When the classroom was being evacuated, more students reported symptoms, and a school-wide alarm was sounded to evacuate the whole school. Around a hundred students and teachers went to the local emergency room, and thirty-eight of them were admitted to the hospital for observation. All medical tests came back negative, and doctors could not find a cause for the reported symptoms. The Environmental Protection Agency conducted an extensive investigation at the school by taking air, water, and wipe samples, and soil gas was analyzed. No source of potential toxins was found.[1] What was going on here? Could these symptoms have been caused by fear of a suspected toxin instead of an actual toxin?

CONCERNS ABOUT
ENVIRONMENTAL HEALTH RISKS

Viewers of the television series *Better Call Saul* may remember the Chuck McGill character, who is convinced that he suffers from a condition called electromagnetic hypersensitivity (EHS). "For reasons unknown, my nervous system has become sensitized to certain frequencies of electromagnetic radiation," as he describes it to a doctor in one of the episodes. "Electronic devices create their own electromagnetic fields. The closer I am to such devices, the worse my symptoms." He goes a long way in protecting himself from these fields by banning all electricity in his home and wearing an aluminum "space blanket."

Although this may be an extreme example, research indicates that between 1.5 and 13.4 percent of the general population in many developed countries report suffering from EHS and attribute health complaints such as headaches and concentration problems to electromagnetic fields from various sources (e.g., mobile phones, power lines).[2] In addition, a large survey showed that around 70 percent of the European population believes that mobile phone towers and high-voltage power lines, both emitting electromagnetic fields (EMFs), affect our health to at least some extent.[3]

When moving from the laboratory or clinical setting into the real world, strictly speaking, we cannot expect "pure" nocebo effects, in the sense of the negative effects of inert treatments on health. In real life we are better off thinking in terms of exposures. Exposures, like EMFs, may or may not to some extent be harmful to our health, depending on the amount of exposure and known toxicity. In some cases, we may be aware that an exposure is bad for our health, such as carbon monoxide from smoking. But in other cases the health effects are still debated and under study. We may have to rely on risk assessment experts and regulatory boards to guide us in what is or isn't safe for our health, and often there is a large amount of uncertainty in their assessments.

Lower-frequency EMFs emitted by mobile phones and high-voltage power lines are good examples of uncertain environmental health risks. It is known that these types of EMFs cannot break bonds between molecules, as opposed to higher-frequency EMFs emitted by sources such as x-rays. As a consequence, there is no direct plausible mechanism for these lower-frequency EMFs to cause cancer.[4] However, epidemiological studies indicate a small but consistent association between exposure to EMFs from high-voltage power lines and childhood leukemia.[5] Some experts interpret the evidence as very weak,[6] while others believe there is at least some reason for concern.[7] With such uncertain risks, it is often difficult to tell to what extent symptoms are caused by environmental exposures and to what extent they are caused by the *perception* of being exposed—that is, the nocebo effect.

Regardless of expert assessments of environmental health risks, people may have concerns about certain environmental exposures, which could lead to nocebo effects. In the scientific literature, research has been conducted into "modern health worries," which refers to perceived risks to personal health from technological change and features of modern life. Such worries tend to cluster around several domains: toxic interventions (e.g., toxic chemicals in household products, poor building ventilation), environmental pollution (e.g., traffic fumes, pesticide spray), tainted food (e.g., genetically modified food, hormones in food), and radiation (e.g., cell phones, high-tension power lines).[8] These concerns are especially prevalent in developed countries but also differ between them. For example, studies show that Swedish people are more concerned about food risks, whereas concern about environmental pollution is more prevalent among New Zealanders.[9] But why are people concerned about these risks? Do these concerns align with expert assessment of the risks? And why does it matter?

THE RISKS OF PERCEIVED EXPOSURE

In the 1980s Paul Slovic and colleagues conducted groundbreaking research in risk perception that may help explain why some risks concern us more than others.[10] By using surveys, they showed that when laypeople judge hazards, they mainly rely on two types of hazard characteristics: first and foremost, the expected dread associated with the risk, and second, how much is known about the risk. A highly dreaded risk is uncontrollable, not equitable, catastrophic, not easily reduced, and involuntary. A highly unknown risk is not observable, it is unknown to those exposed, its effects may be delayed, and its risks are unknown to science. The more dreaded and the more unknown, the higher the perceived risk.

It may then come as no surprise that exposure to EMFs from electric blankets is perceived as less dangerous than exposure to EMFs from high-voltage power lines, even though the actual exposure levels are comparable.[11] Risk perception matters for many areas of research and everyday life—for instance, when studying the link between risk perception and protective behaviors, or when examining communication about risks. But can the perception of being exposed to an environmental risk in itself lead to the experience of symptoms, in line with the examples presented in the previous chapters?

To answer this question, we have to resort to laboratory experiments, as these allow us to rule out effects of the exposure itself. A typical experiment of this sort may look like the following. Imagine you participate in a scientific study aiming to investigate the acute somatic effects of weak to strong EMFs. You are asked to sit on a special seat placed above two large electromagnetic coils, seemingly connected to an impressive power supply. You are told that first you will be exposed to a weak EMF, comparable to everyday exposure, and then to a very strong EMF that is still below the safety norms for EMF exposure. You will have to switch on the power supply yourself and monitor your symptoms during these two episodes.

If you are like the participants in the actual experiment, you will report all sorts of symptoms (such as headaches, dizziness, blurred vision), and to a much larger extent in the second phase, with perceived exposure to the very strong EMF.[12] However, there was a catch. The coils were not actually connected to the machine. No EMFs were emitted during either phase of the study, as this was a sham-exposure study. Similar results were found in another sham-exposure study where participants were supposedly exposed to a new type of EMF to be used in Wi-Fi systems through an antenna mounted on a headband (to bring the signal as close to the body as possible).[13] Again, participants reported more symptoms like headaches and concentration problems after sham exposure.

A similar kind of effect was found in an experimental study conducted in New Zealand on the health effects of infrasound from wind turbines.[14] Infrasound is subaudible low-frequency sound waves emitted by wind turbines, but also by ocean waves, traffic, and various types of machinery. Some people are concerned about the potential health effects of exposure to this type of sound, likely because of information on the internet suggesting negative effects. In a laboratory experiment, participants listened to ten minutes of infrasound from wind turbines and ten minutes of sham infrasound (i.e., no sound) while they received either low-expectancy or high-expectancy information. In the high-expectancy condition, participants saw a video of TV footage containing first-person accounts of side effects attributed to the wind turbines. The low-expectancy condition incorporated a video of TV interviews with experts stating the current scientific position that infrasound produced by wind turbines would not cause symptoms. The researchers did not find a difference in reported symptoms between exposure to the sham infrasound and exposure to the real infrasound. They did, however, find an increase in reported symptoms in those participants who received the high-expectancy information suggesting a link between infrasound and health complaints.

These experiments demonstrate that it is possible to create the experience of symptoms by manipulating perceived exposure to potential environmental risks. But what about real life? We do not live our lives in the controlled setting of laboratory experiments. Being exposed daily to infrasound from a wind turbine close to your home or an EMF from a nearby high-voltage power line is not the same as being voluntarily exposed during a laboratory experiment. In real life we are constantly exposed to all sorts of potential risks and also to information about these risks, while we also manage to perform the daily tasks life asks of us.

NOCEBO RESPONSES TO
HIGH-VOLTAGE OVERHEAD POWER LINES

To properly assess nocebo responses to environmental exposures outside the laboratory, it is important to use a so-called prospective or quasi-experimental design. These kinds of studies are difficult to conduct because one has to know beforehand where and when an exposure is expected to increase. It also requires ample planning and funding. Fortunately, both conditions were met in the Netherlands, where new high-voltage power lines were installed due to increased demand for reliable and sustainable energy and the government provided funding for research on the topic of EMFs and health. This opened up the opportunity for our team to study how people respond when a new source of EMFs is introduced into their environment.

We set up a large-scale study of health responses to the introduction of a new high-voltage power line.[15] Residents living close (0–500 meters) to where a new high-voltage power line was to be installed and a random sample of residents living farther away (500–2,000 meters) were invited to participate in a survey study about their health and the environment. They filled out questionnaires regarding their health and a broad range of environmental factors (including power lines). The first two measurements took place ten and five months before the new line was put into operation. Two more assessments were conducted two and seven months after the line was put into operation. The Dutch transmission system operator communicated with residents when the new line was put into operation.

More than two hundred participants living within 0–300 meters of the new line reported a larger increase in cognitive issues (concentration problems, forgetfulness, etc.) and somatic complaints (headaches, stomachaches, muscle pain, etc.) when compared with the nearly five hundred participants who lived 300–500 meters away and the more than five hundred people who resided 500–2,000 meters away from the line.[16]

As this was not a laboratory study with sham EMF exposure, these results are not direct evidence for a nocebo effect. They do indicate, however, that the installation of a new high-voltage power line may have a negative impact on health perceptions among nearby residents. Although it is unlikely, the results could also be due to increased exposure to EMFs. There is no plausible direct biophysical mechanism for an EMF from power lines to cause the type of health complaints we found in our study at the levels residents were exposed to.[17]

On the other hand, there is quite a bit of evidence for the role of the nocebo effect in triggering acute symptoms in people who describe themselves as sensitive to EMFs.[18] In a follow-up study, we investigated the potential role of nocebo mechanisms to explain the increase in reported symptoms surrounding the new power line.[19] We found that the larger increase in reported symptoms in nearby residents could be explained by the larger increase in the strength of their belief that these symptoms were caused by a power line. This indicates that ideas that residents had about how dangerous a power line would be for their health were related to how dangerous it actually was for their health. This is in line with the previously discussed experimental evidence for nocebo effects from environmental exposures.

When we zoomed in on those residents living within 0–300 meters of the new line, there appeared to be a specific subgroup of residents who became more convinced that their complaints were caused by a high-voltage power line.[20] Before the new line was built, these residents already indicated that they expected to develop health complaints from living close to an overhead power line. They also reported having heard more about the negative health effects of power lines in the media and from friends, and they were more aware of the activation of a new power line in their vicinity. The installation of a new overhead high-voltage power line may have set into motion a process in which ideas and complaints reinforced each other, akin to nocebo effects in experimental studies.

RISK PERCEPTION AND RISK COMMUNICATION

If we want to better understand how to guard ourselves against nocebo responses in our daily lives, we need to understand these processes better. Earlier in this chapter we discussed certain characteristics of a risk that make exposures feel more dangerous (expected dread and how much is known about a risk), regardless of whether experts consider such exposures more dangerous. To some extent these characteristics are determined by the risk itself. Involuntary exposures such as chemical accidents are generally perceived as riskier than voluntary exposures such as taking drugs. But there are other sources as well that influence how we perceive risks. Risk perception takes place in a wider context where hazards and psychological, social, institutional, and cultural factors interact with one another. Communication with others through official and informal personal networks plays a large role. It is not without reason that a whole chapter in this book is devoted to the role of the media in nocebo effects (see Chapter 11). Content analyses of messages in the media regarding the potential health effects of EMFs suggest that these messages are disproportionately negative and not in line with current scientific evidence.[21] Such messages may amplify already existing fears and may eventually lead to nocebo effects, as illustrated by examples discussed in Chapter 11.

To get more insight into these processes, we interviewed residents about their experiences with the planned introduction of a new high-voltage power line near their homes.[22] Countries differ in how they deal with the potential health risks of EMFs from power lines. In the Netherlands the precautionary principle is applied when constructing new power lines. "Better safe than sorry" is the basic idea behind the precautionary principle. This means that power line planners in the Netherlands need to ensure that households and other "sensitive" locations (such as schools and daycare facilities) are not exposed to an average magnetic field strength higher than 0.4 µT (generally < 55 m from the heart of the line), which is suggested as a cutoff value for a higher relative risk of childhood leukemia. If for some households this could not be achieved, residents received an offer to sell their home to the government. We interviewed residents living just outside this mitigation zone.

Interviewed residents acknowledged the large amount of uncertainty regarding health effects of living near a power line; nonetheless, they felt that exposure to EMFs could not be completely harmless. This belief was strengthened by their perceptions of messages in the media and "the word on the street," but also by messages from official authorities regarding EMF risk regulations. Saying there is only a small or nonexistent health risk but at the same time offering certain residents an opportunity to sell their home was perceived as inconsistent, which appeared to amplify health risk perceptions. As one resident said:

> So the uncertainty about how harmful that radiation is, it occasionally comes up in the discussion, but never with a conclusion or anything. . . . I think there's something. I think. But I don't know why, because I'm no expert. But I also think that it can't be a coincidence that they have plans to build the line underground.[23]

Another insight came from residents' experiences with the planning process and with aspects of living near power lines other than EMF exposure. Burdens like the expected visual intrusion and devaluation of property seemed to interact and amplify concern about the health risks of EMFs. As one resident put it:

> We could never buy this house somewhere else. Then you're really talking about different property values than when we started here 30 years ago. . . . Perhaps it's not just the view, although I think it's horrible, but OK, we'll wait and see. But in addition, the fact that for health reasons, it doesn't give you reassurance. Put it another way: what idiot would want to live in a place where you can expect to get ill? I wouldn't know many.[24]

In addition, participants perceived the decision-making process regarding the new line as unfair, leading to feelings of injustice. All these experiences may provoke negative affect, which is tightly linked to experiencing symptoms, as was explained in Part Two of this book.

When we discuss nocebo effects in everyday life, therefore, it is valuable to consider the broader context in which symptoms may occur in response to environmental exposures. There is a body of literature on the topic of psychosocial responses to environmental incidents supporting this point of view.[25] Nocebo effects in daily life not only are about psychological processes within ourselves but also extend into the social and physical environment in which we live. If we want to reduce nocebo responses, we must first acknowledge this fact.

PREVENTING NEGATIVE HEALTH EFFECTS

Because many different factors are involved in producing nocebo responses in our environment, there is not one simple recipe to prevent them from occurring—a topic you've read about in prior chapters. Interestingly, when participants exposed to infrasound from wind turbines reported elevated levels of symptoms in a laboratory study, these symptoms returned to normal levels after researchers offered participants the nocebo effect as an explanation for how infrasound can cause symptoms.[26] This was in contrast to offering a biological explanation, which led to sustained high symptom levels. Education about the nocebo effect may therefore be helpful in reducing nocebo responses.

When translating these findings to real life, it is important to take into account the real-life context. When messages surrounding environmental exposures are communicated in a context of feelings of injustice regarding the planning process, a lack of trust in authorities, and genuine concern about potential health effects, they may increase the outrage already present. Therefore, messages should be tailored to the specific context. When we are concerned about our health it rarely helps if we feel like someone is downplaying those concerns. The key to success may lie in taking concerns seriously by tailoring information to our individual needs and giving honest and full disclosure.

CHAPTER 11

THE NOCEBO EFFECT AND THE MEDIA

Kate MacKrill

A story that involves conflict, violence, or scandal will be front-page news. As Charlotte Blease noted in Chapter 4, in journalism "if it bleeds it leads," often leading to sensationalism. Media stories tend to focus on threats to life or ways of life—that is, war and politics. Another area that receives considerable media attention is health, in particular threats to our health. The news media is a key source of health information for the general public, especially when it involves issues about treatment.[1] Health threats are a go-to media topic. In 2002, news coverage centered on what was subsequently revealed to be an ill-founded link between the measles, mumps, and rubella (MMR) vaccine and autism. Twenty years later, we see a similar pattern with the substantial media focus on the side effects of the COVID-19 vaccine.

Media coverage about the adverse effects of medical treatments is not passively received by audiences. We know that information can influence our expectations, and our expectations can influence our physical experiences, as outlined in previous chapters. For example, a doctor informing a patient about the side effects of a medicine can produce negative symptoms due to the nocebo effect. In a similar vein, reading a CNN article warning about chest pain and breathing problems resulting from the COVID-19 vaccine may induce these symptoms. The only difference between these two situations is the number of people who will potentially be affected—CNN's website has around 500 million visits per month.

It has already been discussed in an earlier chapter how the nocebo effect is responsible for a large proportion of side effects from statin medicines. But is it any coincidence that the reporting rate of muscle pain from statin medicines increased after there was a widespread discussion of this side effect in the media? In March 2007, a Dutch television news program broadcast an item on the serious adverse responses some patients had experienced from statins. In the month before this news item, the Netherlands' adverse reactions monitoring center had received no complaints of statin side effects. After the item aired, there were more than two hundred adverse event reports by patients.[2] The most commonly reported side effect after the news coverage was muscle pain, with muscle weakness and spasms also being prevalent. In this case, the nocebo response was short-lived, as after a couple of weeks the side effect reporting rate returned to the pre–media attention levels.

Some people may be skeptical about media-induced nocebo effects. An alternative explanation to the nocebo effect may be that the media coverage of statin side effects provided a public service by informing patients of the issue and encouraging those who may have been experiencing similar symptoms to report their adverse responses. However, as will be discussed shortly, this explanation doesn't always account for the increase in side effects.

THE VENLAFAXINE BRAND CHANGE

New Zealand has a unique model for the funding of medicines and other medical treatments. The government's pharmaceutical management agency (Pharmac) has a limited budget, which provides the opportunity to negotiate directly with drug companies to market medicines at the lowest possible price. In order to manage its budget, Pharmac often instigates compulsory nationwide switches from a branded version of a particular medicine to its generic equivalent when one becomes available.

In Chapter 1, health psychologists Stefanie Meeuwis and Andrea Evers discussed branded drugs, which are typically the first version of a medicine to appear on the market. To recoup the significant costs of research and development, a branded drug is usually more expensive and is initially under patent, meaning that only the pharmaceutical company that developed it is able to manufacture and sell the medicine. Irrespective of country, patents usually grant the company twenty years of protection starting from the application date. When the patent expires, other companies can produce generic copies of the medicine at a lower cost. Regulatory agencies, such as the U.S. Food and Drug Administration, require generic drugs to be pharmacologically identical to the branded version in order to be approved for use. As Meeuwis and Evers noted, the branded and generic versions of a medicine should have the same efficacy, safety, and side effect profiles. Despite this, generic medicines are often the victim of the nocebo effect, as shown by them being less effective at managing symptoms and having more side effects than the branded version. For example, people perceive the painkiller tramadol to be less effective when it is in generic packaging compared to when they're given the exact same medicine but it's made to look like a branded version.[3] It's also natural for people to dislike change, and so the nocebo effect can come into play when patients are forced to switch from their previous brand to a generic. Past research illustrates that the act of changing medicines usually contributes more to adverse reactions than the actual drug ingredients do.[4] Consequently, these situations readily attract media attention because an increase in side effects following a government-mandated medicine switch is a newsworthy story, which exacerbates nocebo responding even further.

In 2017, Pharmac switched forty-five thousand New Zealanders from their previous brand of the antidepressant venlafaxine to a generic version of the same medicine. There were initial reports on social media that the new generic was not as effective in managing patients' depression and anxiety and was associated with a number of new side effects. These adverse reaction reports prompted a review of the medicine by two separate medicine advisory groups. They concluded that the branded and generic versions were identical and that the increase in side effect complaints was due not to safety or quality issues with the generic medicine but rather to media attention causing a loss of confidence in the medicine.

The impact of media reports on side effects has already been discussed by John Kelley in Chapter 6. Here, I will probe this topic further by highlighting some additional work. In February 2018, two major New Zealand print and online media outlets published articles discussing patients' reports of side effects. Three patients were interviewed who described how the new generic was less effective and caused an increase in various symptoms, including headaches, fatigue, nausea, and, most worryingly, heightened suicidal thoughts. One patient was quoted as saying, "This generic stuff is poison." In April another news article was published that continued the discussion about patients' complaints of side effects. My colleagues and I conducted a study to investigate whether this media coverage would be associated with a subsequent increase in patients' side effect reporting.[5] We analyzed one hundred reports to the New Zealand Centre for Adverse Reactions Monitoring (CARM) and hypothesized that the specific side effects mentioned in the media would show the greatest increase, compared to other side effects that were not mentioned in the coverage but were nevertheless reported at a similar rate prior to the media attention.

In the five months prior to the first media articles in February, patients reported an average of seven side effects per month from the generic venlafaxine. However, in the month directly after the first media articles, sixty-five side effects were reported—an increase in the reporting rate of almost 830 percent. Side effect reporting quickly returned to the pre–media attention average, only to increase by 370 percent following the publication of the second article. In line with our hypothesis, the side effects that were specifically mentioned in the media saw the greatest increase in reports. In particular, suicidal thoughts increased from a monthly average of 0.4 reports to 8 following the first media articles. This may be at least in part a consequence of comments by patients who were interviewed in the newspaper articles, where they reported feeling like they were back in a "dark hole." This type of media reporting is concerning. It is recognized that the reporting of suicide in the media can influence some people's thoughts and behaviors, a phenomenon that has been termed "suicide contagion."[6] As a response, many countries have guidelines for how suicide should be discussed in the media, but this doesn't necessarily extend to the reporting of suicidal thoughts as a side effect of an antidepressant.

In comparison to the symptoms mentioned in the news coverage, the reporting rate of side effects that were not mentioned in the media showed very little change. The media articles also discussed patients' statements that emphasized that the medicine was not working properly. This was mirrored in the CARM reports of reduced drug efficacy, which rose from an average of 4 reports per month to 17 reports following the coverage, an increase of more than 300 percent. This is alarming because the perception that the drug is not effective could potentially cause some people to stop taking their medicine.

But that is not the end of it. Five months on from the print articles, New Zealand's largest television broadcaster aired a series of stories on the venlafaxine brand change in the prime-time news broadcast. The four TV items from September to December 2018 again discussed patients' reports of side effects and noted that more than two hundred people had reported adverse reactions due to the new generic. This provided the opportunity to examine the effect of the television items compared to the print articles on the magnitude of the nocebo effect.[7] We anticipated that the TV coverage would have a greater impact on side effect reporting than the print media reports, but perhaps not to the extent we actually found. Prior to any media coverage, CARM received an average of 7 side effect reports per month for the medicine venlafaxine, as we've noted. After the TV coverage, an average of 236 side effects were reported, with the number of reports reaching a peak of 535 in October. Not only was this greater than the pre–media attention monthly average, but it was also 382 percent greater than the effect of the print articles.

There could be a few explanations for these findings. It could be that the new generic medicine was actually less effective than patients' original version. Or, as mentioned previously, the media coverage might have encouraged people to report their adverse reactions and provided them with a pathway to do so. However, I venture that the most likely explanation for the increase in side effects is a media-induced nocebo effect. The side effects could not be attributed to the ingredients of the drug, as pharmaceutical testing had found the branded and generic formulations to be identical. Additionally, it was the side effects that were specifically mentioned in the media that recorded the greatest change. This suggests that the negative media coverage of the venlafaxine brand change influenced patients' expectations about the generic medicine. These expectations caused patients to pay greater attention to their symptoms and more readily notice side effects in line with their beliefs. Many of the side effects that were mentioned in the media are either symptoms of depression or are commonly experienced in everyday life, such as headaches and fatigue. These could have been misattributed to the generic medicine and reported as side effects. There is a growing body of evidence for the effect of the media in producing nocebo responses. Media reports about side effects have been shown to increase adverse events from other antidepressants,[8] the human papillomavirus vaccine,[9] and levothyroxine,[10] a thyroid replacement medicine. The last example has also demonstrated that the "dosage" of media coverage influences the extent of nocebo responses.

For example, smaller regions where the local newspapers gave more attention to levothyroxine side effects accounted for more adverse event reports than larger cities in which newspapers did not focus on this story.

HOW DOES THE MEDIA PRODUCE
A NOCEBO EFFECT?

What is it about the way the media discusses medicines and side effects that leads to greater nocebo responses? In the age of technology and social media, journalists have to compete with Google and Facebook algorithms to make their articles visible to the desired audience, meaning they purposely select and frame news items to increase "likeability."[11] This is evident in the rise of clickbait articles that attract the audience's attention at the expense of factual reporting. For example, the headline "The Potentially Life-Threatening Side Effects of Taking Statins"[12] has a greater chance of capturing the reader's attention than a more accurate but hypothetical headline such as "Statins Have Significant Benefits, Few Serious Side Effects." The first headline is already molding the reader's expectations about both the story and statin medicines.

This journalistic style is not limited to the headline. There are particular ways that health scares and medicine side effects are discussed in the media that shape expectations and result in nocebo effects. Communication experts have demonstrated how news media can frame a story by selecting certain facts and ignoring or emphasizing particular aspects of a story, which influences how the audience will evaluate the situation. For example, media professionals often interview a few people with specific viewpoints, but generalize these experiences to the wider patient group. This was the case with the newspaper articles on the venlafaxine brand change, which initially included interviews with only three patients but generalized their complaints to the wider patient population. Additionally, later television coverage reported that there were two hundred patient reports of adverse reactions. This statement sounds alarming when taken out of context; however, that number reflects less than 0.5 percent of the total patient group taking venlafaxine (forty-five thousand people). The only difference between these statistics is whether they are reported as an absolute number (the total) or as a relative number (proportion). Reporting such as this can give the audience the impression that a health scare is more prevalent than it actually is and that they are likely to be affected.

Another feature worth noting is the balance—or lack thereof—in media reporting of side effects. In the venlafaxine brand change, there was very little media attention given to medical professionals who claimed that the medicine was safe and effective, and no interviews with patients who switched to the generic medicine without issue (of whom there were thousands). Conversely, balance was artificially created in news stories about the MMR vaccine allegedly causing autism. In the United Kingdom, the media gave equal coverage to both sides of the MMR-autism debate. This led the public to assume there was disagreement in expert opinion when in reality the MMR vaccine had consistently been shown to be safe, effective, and not a cause of autism.[13]

Similarly, the media also frequently reduces the complexity of issues to contrive a sense of conflict. Danish media articles about side effects from antidepressants discussed the topic in a way that implied that pharmaceutical and governmental agencies' financial interests were more important than patients' safety. In the previous ten years, there had been a total of fifty-one reports about antidepressant side effects to the Danish Medicine Agency. In the five months following the discussion of antidepressant side effects in the media, there were thirty-five new reports.[14] It is evident that such reporting can influence the audiences' expectations about the potential health threat of a treatment.

The framing of news stories and interviews with affected patients can result in a process known as social modeling. This occurs when an individual observes another person's response to a treatment and then experiences the same reaction. Studies have cleverly demonstrated how this process occurs. A participant is given some form of treatment, such as a pill or ointment, which in reality is a placebo. The researcher escorts the participant back to a waiting room in order to give the treatment time to "take effect." Here the researcher asks what appears to be a fellow participant how they feel after taking the medicine. This second person is actually a study actor, hired by the researchers, who responds by stating either that they feel fine (no social modeling) or that they are starting to get a headache and feel tired (social modeling present). Studies using this cover story have consistently shown that participants who see another person report side effects go on to report the same symptoms from the placebo treatment compared to those who observed the actor say they felt fine.[15] These studies occur in a very personal setting, with the participant sitting next to the actor in the waiting room, which is likely to create a strong social modeling effect. Nevertheless, the media can produce a similar or even larger social modeling effect, with stories that involve patients discussing treatment side effects having the potential to be seen by thousands of people. It is evident from the venlafaxine studies that people do personally connect with the patients interviewed in the news items. Additionally, it is likely that television media, which allows viewers to see another patient report side effects, results in more impactful social modeling than print, where audiences just read about it.

In 2019 New Zealand's Pharmac switched patients from a branded version of lamotrigine, a medicine for epilepsy and bipolar disorder, to a new generic, and the switch was associated with an increase in side effect complaints. My colleagues and I conducted a lab-based experiment to provide further concrete evidence that the news coverage of this switch was a key factor in influencing side effect reporting.[16] The participants in this study were 108 largely healthy university students who received some information about the lamotrigine switch and were randomly allocated to watch one of three videos. They either saw a real TV news report on the potential side effects from the generic, watched an animated video (made specifically for the study) explaining how the nocebo effect could account for side effects from this medicine, or watched a neutral video explaining how medicines typically work in the body. Participants were informed that the study was testing the short-term mood and cognitive effects of a small dose of lamotrigine. After receiving what they thought to be lamotrigine but was in reality a placebo, we then tracked their side effect reporting and also got them to evaluate the information video they watched.

We found that the group who saw the news item reported a collective total of twenty-eight side effects, while the neutral video group reported sixteen side effects and the nocebo explanation group reported a total of only seven side effects. Participants who watched the news item rated this video as more anxiety-inducing compared to the groups who saw the nocebo explanation or neutral video. In comparison, those who saw our video explaining the nocebo effect found this information about side effects highly reassuring. The advantage of informing patients about the nocebo effect during the side effects disclosure has also been discussed by Mette Sieg and Lene Vase in Chapter 8. This study shows that even though the participants were not actually a patient group taking lamotrigine in real life, they still connected with the patients' stories in the news item. Consequently, participants reported side effects from the placebo tablet and had elevated anxiety because of the news item. This study also investigated whether explaining how the nocebo effect causes side effects could in fact mitigate this process. We showed that simply explaining how the nocebo effect works might help to reduce it. So perhaps the next time a litany of side effects is described in a medicine information leaflet, newspaper article, or TV commercial, it should come with a disclaimer describing the nocebo effect.

WHY DOES THIS MATTER?

Negative media reporting can cause the nocebo effect, and there are countless examples of people experiencing side effects from medical treatments or environmental exposures due to the influence of media coverage on their expectations. Some may see this as no big deal; people often experience side effects from medicines, so what's a few more? However, media-induced nocebo effects can generate not only side effects but also larger consequences. Let's return to statins. In the Dutch study discussed at the beginning of this chapter, not only was there an increase in muscle-related side effects, but 62 percent of patients also stopped taking the statin after watching the news item discussing the medicine's side effects.[17] Other studies have demonstrated that negative media coverage of statin side effects is associated with an increase in heart attacks and cardiac-related deaths because patients stop taking the medicine.[18]

There is a reasonably simple solution to this. Maintaining journalistic freedom is paramount, but this should be balanced against the competing interest of public health and safety. Although the doctor was once the source of all information relating to health and medicine, people now rely on the media for health information. It is not the intent of the media to cause undue harm with their reporting. The media could consult experts on a particular topic to ensure their coverage is a balance of impactful and factual information rather than simply sensational. Media coverage of a medicine switch, for example, could include an explanation of how a switch may affect some patients—allaying rather than arousing fear. If medical treatments were described with more balanced and less emotive language in the media, then it is likely that the unnecessary experience of side effects could be reduced.

CHAPTER 12

FROM GENITAL-SHRINKING PANICS TO HUMMING GIRAFFES

THE MANY DIFFERENT FACES OF THE NOCEBO EFFECT

Robert E. Bartholomew

Under certain conditions men respond as powerfully to fictions as they do to realities, and . . . in many cases they help to create the very fictions to which they respond.
—Walter Lippmann, *Public Opinion*

On June 18, 2002, there was excitement in Nakhon Si Thammarat province in southern Thailand after the discovery of dinosaur fossils in Pedan Cave. Later that month, 15 students in a group of 180 from the Rajabhat Institute who were visiting the site were overcome with dizziness, chest pain, and breathing difficulties. Those affected were rushed to a local exorcist (*mor phi*), and they began to recover after being sprinkled with holy water. Later they were taken to a nearby hospital, where they were examined and released. Several days later, four more students and a teacher from the same institute experienced similar symptoms while leaving the site. This time they were taken to a medical center first, followed by a visit to a local healer who reportedly cast out demons after treating them with more blessed water. Villagers blamed the incidents on spirits guarding the cave and thought that the students' presence might have offended them.[1] In Thai folklore it is widely believed that gravesites like Pedan Cave that hold fossilized remains must be treated with care and respect, as they are often haunted by *phii pob*, spirits that are easily offended. In her study of Thai folklore, Kanya Wattanagun writes that "whimsically picking up a stone, a flower, or any items from a 'sacred area' (a specific part of a forest occupied by forest spirits) can be taken by the offended spirits as a theft that deserves a severe punishment." Illnesses in Thailand are often still attributed to breaking protocols and failing to offer deference to local spirits.[2] As I will explain in this chapter, history is replete with anecdotal accounts of individuals who believed they were the subject of hexes, curses, charms, and spells, which may be instances of the nocebo effect.

THE FALLIBILITY OF THE SENSES

The social, cultural, political, and religious environment of any given person has a powerful effect on how that individual perceives the events and circumstances around them. In 1923, American sociologist William Isaac Thomas famously wrote, "If men define situations as real, they are real in their consequences."[3] What became known as the "Thomas theorem" underscores the idea that beliefs create powerful social realities that can become self-fulfilling. Humans are fallible creatures prone to perceiving the world in ways that differ significantly from reality. Each of our five senses can deceive us. It is well known within the field of criminology that eyewitness testimony is unreliable. This has been borne out in both experimental settings and real life.[4] In the criminal justice system, there are many examples of felons who were convicted on eyewitness testimony and later found innocent. The Innocence Project reports that since 1989, 375 people in the United States have been exonerated using DNA.[5] In popular culture, the fallibility of our senses has given rise to supposed sightings of creatures such as Bigfoot and chupacabras, despite no confirmatory physical evidence.[6]

Our other senses are also fallible. Researchers in psychology and phonetics have found that earwitness testimony is even more unreliable than eyewitness testimony. In summarizing the literature, Helen Fraser found earwitness identification "to be unreliable and misleading," with a potential to contribute to miscarriages of justice within the legal system.[7] A series of tests conducted at the University of Gothenburg involving 949 subjects found that "voice identification under reasonably realistic conditions is a highly difficult task," to the point that many people are unable to even identify the voices of their own family members.[8]

THE IMPORTANCE OF CONTEXT

Humans infer meaning from the world around them. We are motivated to create stories that are personally meaningful and that convey social and psychological importance. Mostly this is an automatic process that happens without our conscious awareness. This has direct relevance to the nocebo effect because psychogenic illness is based on a belief—and all humans have beliefs. What any individual, group, or culture defines as reality is, in part, socially constructed. People order their own versions of reality.[9] Culture is a collection of people who hold similar outlooks and therefore have similar definitions of "reality." Much of this is based not on science but on belief.[10]

What is considered real in one culture or historical period is often seen differently in another. It may be tempting to dismiss non-Western beliefs, such as becoming ill due to a curse or so-called voodoo hexes, because curses are inconsistent with Western medicine and science. The same can be said about the potential pitfalls of using a twenty-first-century lens to evaluate behaviors from earlier eras. Given the variation in human social realities, anyone tempted to pass judgment on beliefs that vary from modern Eurocentric constructions of reality should keep in mind that Western culture has an array of popular social realities with little or no basis in science. These range from the belief that 5G towers spread COVID-19 to the belief of some QAnon adherents that certain American politicians are ritually sacrificing babies. This same culture has a tradition of encouraging children to have false beliefs about the existence of a bearded man in a red suit who delivers presents at Christmas, a giant rabbit who leaves chocolate eggs at Easter, and a fairy who leaves money under pillows in exchange for teeth.

When assessing the possible appearance of nocebo involvement in illness outbreaks across cultures and historical periods, it is essential to understand that these incidents are always situated in unique contexts that render them plausible to the participants. The zeitgeist, or spirit of the times, must be examined.

"EPIDEMICS" OF GENITAL-SHRINKING

Over the past two centuries, there have been several outbreaks of *koro*—a psychiatric term used to describe the perception that one's genitalia are shrinking or retracting into the body. In males, it is most commonly the penis, while in the case of females, victims sometimes believe that their breasts or vulva is shrinking. The term "koro" is believed to have originated from the Malay word *keruk*, meaning "to shrink."[11] The incidence of koro is quite low and usually takes the form of individual cases where the victim is under the social delusion that their genitalia are getting smaller. Of the individual cases that have been recorded, there is a consensus that the victims are typically exhibiting serious psychiatric pathologies such as schizophrenia and depression in conjunction with sexual dysfunction.

These rare cases of koro are commonly viewed as a culture-specific syndrome involving delusions that coincide with acute anxiety, an array of psychosomatic complaints, and a belief in many victims that once the genitalia fully retract or disappear, death will occur. The condition is mostly confined to Asia. The earliest known reference to shrinking or retracting genitalia is in the Chinese medical text *Huangdi Neiching*, which appeared between 200 and 300 BCE. The book describes *suo-yang*, a fatal condition involving the retraction of the penis into the abdomen.[12] There are references to koro in Cantonese-speaking areas (where it is called *sookyong*), Mandarin-speaking regions (*suo-yang*), other parts of mainland China (where it is called *shook yang*, *shook yong*, *suk-yong*, or *so in tchen*), in Sulawesi, Indonesia (*lasa koro*), and in parts of the Philippines (*lannuk e laso*).[13] Koro epidemics have been recorded in China and Singapore, where they were prompted by cultural beliefs, based on long-standing Chinese traditions, that created an expectation of genitalia shrinkage and accompanying symptoms and perceptions. In each of these episodes, the most important factor shaping the nocebo experience was plausibility, which was in turn shaped by the context.

"EPIDEMICS" OF *KORO* IN CHINA AND SINGAPORE

Between November 1984 and May 1985, more than two thousand inhabitants in an isolated region of Guangdong, China, were swept up in a genital-shrinking panic. Many inhabitants believed that the spirits of female fox spirits wander the countryside in search of penises to steal.[14] Of 232 patients surveyed, all expressed the belief that female fox spirits could cause *suo-yang*. Most of the "attacks" took place at night, with the victim experiencing a chilly sensation followed by a feeling that their penis was shrinking.[15] An eighteen-year-old agriculture student provided the following account during the outbreak:

> I woke up at midnight and felt sore and numb in my genitals. I felt . . . [my penis] was shrinking, disappearing. I yelled for help, my family and neighbours came and held my penis. They covered me with a fish net and beat me with branches of a peach tree. . . . The peach tree branches are the best to drive out ghosts or devils. They said they'd catch the ghost in the net. They were also beating drums and setting off firecrackers. . . . They had to repeat the procedure until I was well again, until the ghost was killed by the beating.[16]

During the episode, several children reported shrinkage of their nose, ears, and tongue. This reflects the prevalent ancient Chinese belief that any male (yang) organ can shrink or retract, with protruding body parts such as the penis, breasts, nipples, tongue, nose, hands, feet, and ears being yang.[17] A separate "epidemic" in 1987 affected at least three hundred residents in the vicinity of Haikang town on the Leizhou peninsula of Guangdong province.[18] Koro is endemic in parts of southern China, with sporadic annual reports and occasional case clusters. Epidemics involving at least several hundred people have been documented since the mid-1800s.[19]

The wider cultural context is the key to understanding these episodes. In parts of China, koro is a taken-for-granted reality that can result from an imbalance of the yin and yang forces. It is believed that the shrinkage can occur when the yin dominates the yang.[20] Curative or preventive measures include applying or consuming yang elements (e.g., consuming ginger, red pepper jam, or black pepper powder, or tying a yam stem around the penis).[21]

SONIC SCARES: HAVANA SYNDROME

In November 2016, two U.S. intelligence officers working in a small station in Havana, Cuba, began noticing mysterious high-pitched sounds near their homes at night. On December 30, one of the officers developed a headache, ear pain, and hearing problems and sought treatment at the American embassy clinic. During his exam he wondered if there might be a connection between his symptoms and a beam of sound that appeared to be directed at his home at night. Embassy officials then learned that two other officers working in the same field office had reported similar sounds outside their homes the previous month, and a theory emerged that the agents were being harassed by a new weapon that used sound waves to make victims sick. Incidents of the condition, which was eventually dubbed "Havana Syndrome," were confined to one of two hotels, an apartment complex, and diplomats' homes. Word of the "attacks" spread quickly through the American and Canadian embassies, which had been sharing intelligence. By April 2017, U.S. embassy officials began advising staff to avoid standing or sleeping near windows. Such advisories would have been alarming and stressful, especially for those with children. As one embassy staffer told me, once word of the "attacks" got out, "many of us were experiencing headaches, mental fog, irritability, etc.," which was "completely un-derstandable given the high stress environment and the fact that we went asleep every night wondering whether we'd be zapped in our beds, and consequently lay awake for hours at a time, days on end, stretching into weeks and months."[22]

THE HISTORICAL BACKDROP AND
SENSATIONAL MEDIA COVERAGE

Episodes of social contagion are always couched in a unique context that renders the perceived threat to be plausible and imminent. In the case of Havana Syndrome, lingering political animosities were pivotal to instilling fear, as the Trump administration interpreted the events as a continuation of Cold War hostilities. Prior to their posting, the diplomats had been briefed on the aggressive history of harassment by Cuban agents and the likelihood of twenty-four-hour surveillance. In the past, Cuban operatives would sneak into homes and rearrange bookshelves and furniture, leave cigarette butts, and open windows as a way of conveying to the residents that they were being watched. The State Department's inspector general has documented several harassing actions by Cuban agents, ranging "from the petty to the poisoning of family pets."[23] Havana Syndrome was only identified as a health issue in February 2017. Soon diplomats being posted to Havana were being told that they might be the next target of a sonic weapon and were played recordings of the "attack" made by their colleagues. The counseling of new staff created an expectation of illness—that is, a nocebo effect—and with it, a frame through which future sounds and symptoms were interpreted.

In December 2020, a National Academy of Sciences panel suggested that the most likely explanation for the "attacks" was pulsed microwave radiation, with the microwaves stimulating a nerve in the inner ear that resulted in the perception of a barely discernible clicking. In September 2021, a classified government report was released revealing that of the first twenty-one "attack" victims, eight had made audio recordings. This ruled out microwaves as the culprit because it is not possible to make an audio recording of microwaves. Microwaves would also interfere with electronics and knock out Wi-Fi, and none of that was reported in Cuba. The investigators concluded that the recordings were consistent with the mating call of the Indies short-tailed cricket.[24]

Media coverage of the episode also served to crystallize the belief that something nefarious was afoot, with reports of changes in the brain's white matter, brain damage, and hearing loss—each subsequently proved to be wrong. In December 2017 doctors examining a cohort of embassy patients leaked information that they had found white matter changes in their brains. After thirteen months of media speculation, in February 2018 a study published in the

Journal of the American Medical Association found "nonspecific white matter changes" in three of twenty-one patients.[25] This finding was unremarkable because white matter changes are common in a number of conditions ranging from migraines to depression to normal aging. A 2019 study in the same journal found brain anomalies in a group of embassy diplomats, prompting dramatic headlines about brain damage. However, brain changes are not the same as brain damage. It is not unusual to find minor anomalies in small cohorts. Similar anomalies can be caused by exposure to prolonged stress. Significantly, twelve of the affected diplomats had a history of concussion, and none of the healthy controls did. This alone could account for the differences between the groups.[26]

A GLOBAL EXPERIMENT IN MASS SUGGESTION

Once the State Department established it was likely that members of their diplomatic corps in Cuba had been attacked, intelligence officers and diplomatic staff stationed around the world were warned to be vigilant for "anomalous health incidents" associated with strange sounds that had been experienced over the previous several years. In September 2021 the Department of Defense (DOD) issued a similar alert to its 2.9 million service members and contractors. Defense secretary Lloyd Austin wrote, "Over the course of the last several years, and predominantly overseas, some DOD . . . personnel have reported a series of sudden and troubling sensory events such as sounds, pressure, or heat concurrently or immediately preceding the sudden onset of symptoms such as headaches, pain, nausea, or disequilibrium (unsteadiness or vertigo)."[27] Sociologists refer to this as a "self-fulfilling prophecy," reminiscent of the old adage "Speak of the devil and he is bound to appear." Unsurprisingly, by early 2022, as U.S. officials began to redefine an array of health conditions under a new label, more than a thousand reports of "attacks" outside Cuba had been received in over a dozen countries from Australia to Uzbekistan.

In 2019, "energy attacks" were reported by U.S. officials working in and near the White House. Closer scrutiny of these reports suggests the appearance of common neurological conditions involving part of the inner ear that is responsible for balance and spatial awareness.[28] Once you eliminate the claims of brain damage and hearing loss, you are left with an array of vague symptoms: headache, nausea, dizziness, fatigue, difficulty concentrating, confusion, disorientation, forgetfulness, insomnia, tinnitus, balance problems, ear pain and pressure, nosebleeds, and depression. These symptoms are so common that nearly everyone would experience some of them in any given week of their life.

The vague nature of the symptoms, the absence of any identifiable weapon, and the physical limitations of sonic or microwave weapons all point to a nocebo effect along with the redefinition of a variety of ailments that have been placed under the category "Havana Syndrome." State Department officials failed to realize that the involvement of four people from the same CIA station strongly suggested mass psychogenic illness, which is known to follow social networks. Outbreaks commonly begin in small, cohesive units and spread outward, starting with people of higher status. In the Havana case, those affected belonged to a common work environment and social network, were under extreme stress in a foreign country where they knew they were under constant surveillance, and were then told they might be the targets of a sonic weapon.

Which of the following is more likely—that American and Canadian diplomats stationed in Cuba were the target of a mysterious new weapon that defies the laws of physics, or that they were experiencing symptoms generated by the nocebo effect, a well-known phenomenon that has been described for millennia, albeit under an array of different names? The weight of evidence supports the latter explanation. In January 2022 the contents of an ongoing CIA investigation into the episode were made public. An analysis of more than a thousand cases of "anomalous health incidents" that were considered to be potential attacks concluded that all but a small fraction of reports were explainable from mundane causes such as anxiety or preexisting health conditions. As for the small number of cases listed as unexplained, there was insufficient data with which to render an assessment.[29] This is not unlike past U.S. government investigations into the origin of unidentified flying objects; just because a case is classified as "unexplained" does not necessarily mean it is evidence for the existence of space aliens traversing the skies. Similarly, the presence of unfamiliar sounds coinciding with health complaints cannot be taken as confirmation of a secret energy weapon. In the case of Havana Syndrome, it would be wise to consider the old medical adage: "When you hear the sound of hoofbeats in the night, first think horses, not zebras."

FROM HUMMING GIRAFFES TO
THE GLASS ARMONICA

Claims of sonic weapons causing ill health in Cuba are reminiscent of more recent scares involving wind turbines and giraffes. In 2016, it was discovered that giraffes communicate using infrasound that emanates from the two outcroppings on their heads known as ossicones. Soon after media reports of this finding appeared, residents living near the giraffe enclosure at the Paignton Zoo in Bristol, England, became convinced that the animals were making them sick. In all, 165 people signed a petition complaining that they were suffering from a variety of ailments ranging from insomnia and tremors to headaches, heart palpitations, and irritation. One resident, Gillian Watling, said that at night the noise created "waves passing down the muscles in my back, buttocks, thighs and calves." While residents claimed that they could hear a mysterious humming sound, the local council dispatched officers to the enclosure but were unable to detect any unusual sounds and even ruled out the possibility of low-frequency noise from a nearby factory. One of the researchers in the giraffe study noted that not only was the hum barely audible, at 92 Hz, but after monitoring the animals for nine hundred hours, there were only sixty-five incidents of giraffe hums, none of which lasted for more than a few seconds.

In Chapter 10, psychologist Jarry Porsius described the relationship between nocebo effects and wind turbines. Even earlier, one of the most remarkable episodes involving claims of sound and health occurred during the eighteenth century and involved one of America's most iconic political figures. During the later seventeenth and early eighteenth centuries, it was widely believed that listening to the strains of certain instruments could adversely affect the nervous system through overstimulation. Women were considered to be particularly vulnerable due to their "weak constitutions." A typical view of the period was expressed by influential Irish physician James Johnson, who in 1837 asserted that music was detrimental to the "delicate" female nervous system. He wrote: "The mania for music injures the health and even curtails the life of thousands and tens of thousands annually, of the fair sex."[30] Music historian James Kennaway observes that the widespread association between music and health may have a psychological origin: "It should also be remembered that it is quite possible that many of the accounts of music causing disease refer to real physical symptoms and suffering, albeit generally with a psychosomatic rather than direct physiological explanation."[31]

One instrument, the glass harp, stands out for its reputed placebo properties during this period. During the late 1700s there were many performers who toured Europe giving concerts with the harp, which was composed of "musical glasses" filled with varying amounts of water. When the rim of each glass was rubbed with a wet finger or tapped with a stick, it produced different tones. Psychologist Stanley Finger observes that during this period many audience members claimed that the sounds had curative effects.[32]

After being inspired by watching a concert with musical glasses, in 1761 American statesman Benjamin Franklin invented an instrument that created high-pitched musical notes by using moistened fingers to touch spinning glass discs of various circumferences. This instrument, the glass armonica, became so popular that Beethoven, Mozart, and Strauss all wrote compositions for the instrument. It was soon being played in concert halls across North America and Europe amid claims that its music, like that of its predecessor, had therapeutic properties. Correspondingly, many audience members reported being healed of various ailments. One illustration of this is detailed in the memoir of Polish princess Izabela Czartoryska, who met Franklin in 1772 and claimed to have had her health restored after he played for her: "I was ill, in a state of melancholia, and writing my testament and farewell letters. . . . Surprised by my immobility, he [Franklin] took my hands and gazed at me saying: *pauvre jeune femme*. He then opened a harmonium, sat down and played long. The music made a strong impression on me and tears began flowing from my eyes. Then Franklin sat by my side and looking with compassion said, 'Madam, you are cured.'"[33]

Then something curious happened. Two prominent armonica players fell ill, prompting rumors that the device was harmful. Before long, instead of reporting improved health, concertgoers began reporting an array of complaints. By the 1780s, shifting popular sentiments had transformed the armonica from a placebo to a nocebo. One of the leading drivers of the scare was German composer Karl Röllig, an armonica player who wrote an essay in 1787 in which he alarmingly claimed that listening to it for too long could induce not only various ailments but death. He offered himself as an example and claimed that his playing the instrument had triggered a number of health issues, from tremors and muscle spasms to dizziness and visions—which he said stopped when he ceased playing.[34] Amid accounts of its deleterious effects on human health, the armonica waned in popularity by the end of the century.

Whether it is genital-shrinking panics or claims of sound causing health complaints, the role of the nocebo effect has had a significant impact throughout history. These cases demonstrate the importance of examining the social, cultural, and historical backdrop and its role in framing nocebo-based illness outbreaks. It is important to acknowledge that the belief that illness can result from a plethora of causes that have no scientific grounding is common around the globe. Beliefs in curses, hexes, "root work," and so on are widespread. They should not necessarily be viewed as examples of abnormality or dysfunction. These episodes involve people who are trying to make sense of their world. In April 1976 fifteen girls at the Sand Flat School in Mount Pleasant, Mississippi, began to act strangely. They would scream, collapse, and roll around on the floor. Some appeared to lose consciousness or began calling out while in a trancelike state. Some students yelled, "Don't let it get me!" or "Get it off!" before passing out. While it was initially assumed that the pupils were high on drugs, tests were negative. A popular folk theory among parents held that "voodoo spells" were to blame and that one of the affected girls had been hexed by a rival classmate in a bid to gain the romantic affections of a boy. After the first few girls were afflicted, the fear of "black magic" quickly spread through the rest of the group, serving to confirm the reality of the "attack." In an apparent reference to the possible use of "voodoo dolls," one of the affected girls said, "My head was hurting bad. It wasn't like a headache. It felt like something was sticking in it. . . . I couldn't get enough air. Then I fell out—fainted."[35]

We need to be cautious in passing judgment on those who have convictions that differ from mainstream thought. There is a remarkable spectrum of beliefs, many of which have no grounding in science. Outbreaks will continue to be a challenge for health professionals, especially in the age of mass electronic communication, which has transformed our world into a global village as rumors and misinformation travel around the globe in the blink of an eye—or the post of a TikTok video. While we may be living in the twenty-first century with an expanded scientific tool kit, in some respects those who have investigated similar outbreaks in previous centuries had one advantage over the modern era—they did not have to contend with the spread of rumors and unvetted claims on social media, which typically exacerbates episodes. No one is immune from the nocebo effect, because the fundamental component of any outbreak is a belief—and we all have beliefs.

CONCLUSION

Michael H. Bernstein, Charlotte Blease,
Cosima Locher, and Walter A. Brown

NOCEBOS AND EXPECTATIONS

In 1962, Dr. Yujiro Ikemi and Dr. Shunji Nakagawa from the Institute of Psychosomatic Medicine in Japan published an interesting paper.[1] They began by noting, with some skepticism, that people had reported developing an allergic reaction to a lacquer tree from merely walking under one or passing in front of a factory that used the trees as raw material for furniture making. Ikemi and Nakagawa were skeptical that the lacquer tree really caused such severe allergic reactions and pointed out that prior reports had failed to study the phenomenon from "the psychosomatic standpoint." They took several boys fifteen to eighteen years old and touched their skin with either leaves from a chestnut tree, which are not known to cause any sort of allergic reaction, or leaves from a lacquer tree. However, the boys were frequently deceived—thinking, for example, that either the lacquer leaf was the harmless chestnut leaf or the chestnut leaf was actually the lacquer leaf. Having now read all about the nocebo effect, you might predict what happened next. In many cases, the subjects responded in a manner consistent with what they *believed* they were touching. For instance, one boy who had a severe lacquer allergy was touched on his left arm with a chestnut leaf but told it was a lacquer leaf. After twenty minutes, his left arm started "flushing." After fifty minutes, redness, swelling, and blisters appeared.

It can be tempting to dismiss these kinds of stories as one-off instances of people who are gullible, anxious, or unsophisticated. But it is surprisingly easy for anyone to fall prey to nocebo effects, even an editor of this book.

In the summer of 2022, one of us (Bernstein) tested positive for COVID-19, and before long he had all the usual symptoms—fever, congestion, nausea, and fatigue. His doctor prescribed a five-day course of Paxlovid, an antiviral medication used to treat COVID, and he quickly began feeling better. However, he was warned about a rebound effect, in which symptoms return when you're finished taking the medicine. At the time, we were deep in the throes of editing this book, and so nocebo effects were very much on our minds. As you might imagine, Bernstein winced when he heard that warning, worried that now his COVID symptoms would rebound because he expected them to. Sure enough, the day after finishing Paxlovid, he woke up feeling lousy. Nocebo effects may well have played a role.

AS YOU CAN SEE IN THE PRIOR CHAPTERS, data from laboratories and clinics consistently support the notion that information about what to expect has a profound effect on what we experience. If you read about the nocebo effect from an article in the popular press, you'll probably hear about patients enrolled in a clinical trial who experience side effects even though they are actually receiving a placebo. And this certainly does occur, as covered in some of the chapters. But the nocebo effect comprises much more than this important yet narrow example. Nocebo effects are common-place because, as we discussed in the introduction, *expectations are all around us*. The nocebo effect can be invoked if a medical provider is not careful in the way he communicates with a patient. A doctor, nurse, or psychotherapist can rather easily convey negative expecta-tions to patients.

But you can experience a nocebo effect without even stepping foot into an office. It can arise as the result of encountering any negative health expectation, and the consequences can be large. In early 2023, a group of researchers led by Siddhartha Roy looked at data from 2011 to 2019 and proposed that the nocebo effect may even have played a role in the Flint water crisis.[2] As American read-ers will remember, the Flint water crisis was a major scandal in 2014 after water in the city of Flint, Michigan, was found to have been contaminated with lead. Parents, teachers, and members of the pub-lic were understandably concerned about how this would harm the intellectual development of children. The onset of the water cri-sis did in fact coincide with a worsening of educational outcomes, with more students entering special education. However, and this is the critical part, the percent of children with an elevated blood lead level in Flint was always lower than the nearby city of Detroit, Michigan, and almost always lower than the state of Michigan as a whole. Furthermore, while there was indeed a temporary increase in the number of Flint children with an elevated lead rate during the worst of the water crisis, the overall trend over the course of several years was a substantial reduction.

What do we think caused the children to perform worse at school? Was it the water? Or might it have been the fact that, as the researchers put it, "several teachers openly expressed their belief that Flint children had been brain damaged, were incapable of learning, and that there was little point in trying to teach them"?

So what can be done to reduce these unwanted effects? Specific strategies were discussed in several chapters. Perhaps the best approach is the most straightforward: providers should be taught about the nocebo effect. We realize that medical education is already densely packed and adding more material to the curriculum is no easy feat. But even one or two seminars discussing the nocebo effect and the importance of expectation would be advisable. If doctors' first duty is to "do no harm," then it only follows that they should be taught about harms from the nocebo effect and ways of preventing it.

NOCEBO EFFECTS CAN BE VIEWED as a special case of the broader phenomenon of expectations—what we think will happen impacting what actually does happen. While nocebo effects relate to medical outcomes, the role of expectations is actually a much broader phenomenon. In one classic study from the early 1970s, Alan Marlatt and colleagues asked thirty-two men with alcoholism to take part in a taste test.[3] They were asked to sample a variety of either alcoholic or nonalcoholic drinks for fifteen minutes. But there was a catch. Half of the time the subjects were truthfully informed about what they were drinking, while the other half of the time they were told the opposite. According to one important theory of alcoholism at the time, *regardless of what they were told*, the men who were given an alcoholic drink would "lose control" due to the physiological effect of alcohol and consume much more of the drink than the men who were given the non-alcoholic drink.

As it turned out, the drink itself did not matter. What mattered was what participants *believed they were drinking*. During the taste test, more than twice as much of the nonalcoholic drink was consumed when the participants were falsely told it was alcoholic versus when they were truthfully told it was nonalcoholic. Furthermore, more than twice as much alcohol was consumed when participants were honestly told the drink was alcoholic versus when they were falsely told it was nonalcoholic. This study is a powerful demonstration of the role of expectation.

Another example comes from the relatively recent use of "trigger" or "content" warnings in colleges. Content warnings alert a student to the fact she is about to see something unpleasant that could cause anxiety, fear, or other negative emotions. Content warnings are predicated on the admirable goal of protecting people when exposing them to disturbing material. And it is certainly true that books, lectures, or PowerPoint presentations can at times be disturbing given one's personal history. A victim of sexual assault may be flooded with memories of an attack when reading about rape statistics in a criminology course. A student whose best friend died of a fentanyl overdose may be overwhelmed with rage when learning in a neuroscience class about how opioids become addictive.

So before such material is presented, why not offer a trigger warning—telling students that they are about to read something that might be upsetting? You can probably see the parallel to what's been discussed in this book. Trigger warnings may instill negative expectations. And indeed, studies in which students are assigned to either see or not see a trigger warning prior to viewing troubling material have shown that such warnings are not effective in reducing anxiety.[4] In some cases they may even be countertherapeutic.[5]

WHERE DO WE GO FROM HERE?

The authors of the preceding chapters were thorough in covering relevant studies that have been published to date. Still, this book is hardly the last word on the nocebo effect. Many questions remain, and we should focus our attention on answering them.

Many times, nocebo effects are thought of as conscious experiences. If a doctor tells you that a drug may cause an upset stomach, and you think, "This is the last thing I need before my office Christmas party," your doctor evoked a *conscious* expectation. But that's not always how it happens, and we don't yet know the degree to which nocebo is a conscious versus subconscious experience. The way people amplify or misattribute symptoms, as John Kelley explained, is typically outside conscious awareness. The role of consciousness in nocebo effects should be explored more than it has been.

The topic of how to manage the nocebo effect is also underexamined. Several chapters in this volume tackle this important issue, discussing what doctors and other health professionals can do to diminish nocebo effects. Clever strategies have been proposed, such as reducing the amount of side effect information, authorized concealment, and positive framing. We also discuss medical education above. However, despite the importance of this issue there is a serious lack of relevant data. There have been very few careful studies of the proposed approaches to nocebo mitigation. Those that have been done are small and require replication.[6] Relatedly, we really have almost no data from empirical studies on what patients can do. In Chapter 9, Wayne Jonas and Steve Bierman drew on their extensive clinical experience to come up with some intriguing ideas. These should be tested, and such research would be ripe for collaboration between academics and patients.

Finally, as more data on the nocebo effect come in, we can start figuring out which groups are especially likely to experience a nocebo effect and respond to nocebo reduction strategies. Are men different from women in this respect? What about differences by race, socioeconomic status, personality traits, education, or geographic region? Thoughtful investigations of these topics can allow for targeted, evidence-based approaches to reduce nocebo effects.[7]

THE NEXT TIME YOU SEE A CLINICIAN, you might find yourself paying special attention to what she is saying and how that impacts your expectations of the visit. If this does happen, then we have done our job in assembling a relevant and engaging compendium of chapters on the nocebo effect.

Health, vitality, and well-being are all critical. As a society, we invest considerable sums in state-of-the-art facilities to develop new treatments and cures. We mandate that physicians undergo years of intensive training in biology, anatomy, and chemistry before they can treat a patient unsupervised. But as mundane as it sounds, mere language is important too. Words can make us sick. Let's choose them carefully.

ACKNOWLEDGMENTS

We thank our agent, Jessica Papin, for her unwavering support of this project. Daniela Rapp of Mayo Clinic Press was enthusiastic about the book from the beginning and has been a delight to work with. We thank the chapter authors for their patience and dedication to this project, even when "one more draft" was more wishful thinking than reality. Charlotte Blease's late partner, Henry McDonald, gave support to this book and generously offered to provide a patient perspective on some of the ideas presented within it.

All editors have been supported by a strong network of family and friends. We are indebted to them for their support, guidance, love, and encouragement. You know who you are. Thank you.

LIST OF CONTRIBUTORS

Marco Annoni, Ph.D.
Bioethicist, Interdepartmental Center for Research Ethics and Integrity, National Research Council of Italy

Robert E. Bartholomew, Ph.D.
Honorary Senior Lecturer, Department of Psychological Medicine, University of Auckland, New Zealand

Michael H. Bernstein, Ph.D.
Assistant Professor, Department of Diagnostic Imaging, Warren Alpert Medical School of Brown University, Providence, Rhode Island, USA

Steve Bierman, M.D.
Fellowship Faculty, Andrew Weil University of Arizona Center for Integrative Medicine, Tucson, USA

Maxie Blasini, M.S.
California Regional Program Manager, Healthy Food in Health Care, Health Care Without Harm, San Diego, California, USA

Charlotte Blease, Ph.D.
Researcher, Digital Psychiatry, Beth Israel Deaconess Medical Center, Harvard Medical School, Boston, USA, and Department of Women's and Children's Health, Uppsala University, Uppsala, Sweden

Walter A. Brown, M.D.
Clinical Professor Emeritus, Department of Psychiatry and Human Behavior, Warren Alpert Medical School of Brown University, Providence, Rhode Island, USA

Luana Colloca, M.D., Ph.D., M.S.
MPower Distinguished Professor and Director, Placebo Beyond Opinions Center, School of Nursing, University of Maryland, Baltimore, USA

Andrea W. M. Evers, Ph.D.
Professor of Health Psychology and Scientific Director at the Institute of Psychology of Leiden University; Medical Delta Professor at Leiden University, Technical University Delft, and Erasmus University, Rotterdam, The Netherlands

Wayne B. Jonas, M.D.
*President of Healing Works Foundation
Clinical Professor of Family Medicine, Georgetown University School of Medicine, Washington, DC, USA*

John M. Kelley, Ph.D.
Deputy Director, Program in Placebo Studies, Harvard Medical School Distinguished Professor of Psychology, Endicott College, Beverly, Massachusetts, USA

Helen Koechlin, Ph.D.
Senior Researcher at the Division of Psychosomatics and Psychiatry at the University Children's Hospital Zurich of the University of Zurich, Switzerland

Cosima Locher, Ph.D.
Senior Researcher at the Department of Consultation-Liaison Psychiatry and Psychosomatic Medicine at the University Hospital Zurich of the University of Zurich, Switzerland

Kate MacKrill, Ph.D., PGDip Health Psych
Health Psychologist at Te Whatu Ora—Health New Zealand and Honorary Research Fellow in the Department of Psychological Medicine, Faculty of Medical and Health Sciences, University of Auckland, New Zealand

Stefanie H. Meeuwis, Ph.D.
Postdoctoral Researcher at the Health, Medical and Neuropsychology Unit of the Institute of Psychology of Leiden University and at the Institute of Psychology, Jagiellonian University, Kraków, Poland

Jarry T. Porsius, Ph.D.
Senior Researcher at PBL Netherlands Environmental Assessment Agency

Giordana Segneri, M.A.
Assistant Dean for Marketing and Communications, School of Nursing, University of Maryland, Baltimore, USA

Mette Sieg, M.Sc.
Ph.D. fellow at Division for Psychology and Neuroscience, Department of Psychology and Behavioral Science, Aarhus University, Denmark

Lene Vase, Ph.D., DMSc.
Professor, Psychology and Neuroscience, Department of Psychology and Behavioral Science, Aarhus University, Denmark

NOTES

INTRODUCTION

1. "COVID-19 Coronavirus Pandemic," Worldometer, last updated April 25, 2023, Worldometers.info/coronavirus.
2. "More Than 12.7 Billion Shots Given: Covid-19 Tracker," Bloomberg, last updated October 6, 2022, https://www.bloomberg.com/graphics /covid-vaccine-tracker-global-distribution/.
3. *The Reports of the Royal Commission of 1784 on Mesmer's System of Animal Magnetism and Other Contemporary Documents*, translated by I. M. L. Donaldson (Edinburgh: James Lind Library and Sibbald Library, Royal College of Physicians of Edinburgh, 2014), https://www.rcpe.ac.uk/sites /default/files/files/the_royal_commission_on_animal_-_translated_by_iml _donaldson_1.pdf.
4. H. S. Diehl, "Medicinal Treatment of the Common Cold," *Journal of the American Medical Association* 101, no. 26 (1933): 2042–2049, doi:10.1001 /jama.1933.02740510034009.
5. H. S. Diehl, A. B. Baker, and D. W. Cowan, "Cold Vaccines: A Further Evaluation," *Journal of the American Medical Association* 115, no. 8 (1940): 593–594, doi:10.1001/jama.1940.02810340021007.
6. S. Wolf and R. H. Pinsky, "Effects of Placebo Administration and Occurrence of Toxic Reactions," *Journal of the American Medical Association* 155, no. 4 (1954): 339–341, doi:10.1001/jama.1954 .03690220013004.
7. H. K. Beecher, "The Powerful Placebo," *Journal of the American Medical Association* 159, no. 17 (1955): 1602–1609, doi:10.1001/jama .1955.02960340022006.
8. S. Bokat-Lindell, "Is 'Havana Syndrome' an 'Act of War' or 'Mass Hysteria'?," *New York Times*, October 26, 2021.
9. L. Jakes, "Cases of 'Havana Syndrome' Reported at U.S. Embassy in Colombia," *New York Times*, October 12, 2021.
10. S. Schmemann, "The Mystery of 'Havana Syndrome,'" *New York Times*, November 3, 2021.
11. "Why Are Americans Paying More for Healthcare?," Peter G. Peterson Foundation, January 30, 2023, https://www.pgpf.org/blog/2023/01 /why-are-americans-paying-more-for-healthcare.

12. I. Papanicolas, L. R. Woskie, and A. K. Jha, "Health Care Spending in the United States and Other High-Income Countries," *Journal of the American Medical Association* 319, no. 10 (2018): 1024–1039, doi:10.1001/jama.2018.1150.

13. P. Vankar, "Annual Medical Care Price Inflation Rate in the U.S. from 2000 to 2022," Statista, October 18, 2022, https://www.statista.com/statistics/1337585/medical-care-price-inflation-rate-in-the-us/.

14. M. A. Makary and M. Daniel, "Medical Error—The Third Leading Cause of Death in the US," *BMJ* 353 (2016): i2139, doi:https://doi.org/10.1136/bmj.i2139.

15. J. H. Watanabe, T. McInnis, and J. D. Hirsch, "Cost of Prescription Drug–Related Morbidity and Mortality," *Annals of Pharmacotherapy* 52, no. 9 (2018): 829–837, doi:10.1177/1060028018765159.

16. J. C. Vereen and M. Weiss, "Trends in Emergency Hospital Admissions in England Due to Adverse Drug Reactions: 2008–2015," *Journal of Pharmaceutical Health Services Research* 8, no. 1 (2017): 5–11, https://doi.org/10.1111/jphs.12160.

17. W. N. Insani, C. Whittlesea, H. Alwafi, K. K. C. Man, S. Chapman, and L. Wei, "Prevalence of Adverse Drug Reactions in the Primary Care Setting: A Systematic Review and Meta-Analysis," *PLoS One* 16, no. 5 (2021): e0252161, doi:10.1371/journal.pone.0252161.

18. G. C. Alexander, M. Tajanlangit, J. Heyward, O. Mansour, D. M. Qato, and R. S. Stafford, "Use and Content of Primary Care Office-Based vs Telemedicine Care Visits During the COVID-19 Pandemic in the US," *JAMA Network Open* 3, no. 10 (2020): e2021476, doi:10.1001/jamanetworkopen.2020.21476.

CHAPTER 1: THE NOCEBO EFFECT IN THE CLINIC

1. A. Gupta, D. Thompson, A. Whitehouse, T. Collier, B. Dahlof, N. Poulter, R. Collins, and P. Sever, "Adverse Events Associated with Unblinded, but Not with Blinded, Statin Therapy in the Anglo-Scandinavian Cardiac Outcomes Trial-Lipid-Lowering Arm (ASCOT-LLA): A Randomised Double-Blind Placebo-Controlled Trial and Its Non-Randomised Non-Blind Extension Phase," *Lancet* 389, no. 10088 (2017): 2473–2481, doi:10.1016/s0140-6736(17)31075-9.

2. N. Mondaini, P. Gontero, G. Giubilei, G. Lombardi, T. Cai, A. Gavazzi, and R. Bartoletti, "Finasteride 5 mg and Sexual Side Effects: How Many of These Are Related to a Nocebo Phenomenon?," *Journal of Sexual Medicine* 4, no. 6 (2007): 1708–1712, doi:10.1111/j.1743-6109.2007.00563.x.

3. P. E. Penson, G. B. J. Mancini, P. P. Toth, S. S. Martin, G. F. Watts, A. Sahebkar, D. P. Mikhailidis, and M. Banach, "Introducing the 'Drucebo' Effect in Statin Therapy: A Systematic Review of Studies Comparing Reported Rates of Statin-Associated Muscle Symptoms, Under Blinded

and Open-Label Conditions," *Journal of Cachexia, Sarcopenia, and Muscle* 9, no. 6 (2018): 1023–1033, doi:10.1002/jcsm.12344.

4. A. Skvortsova, D. S. Veldhuijzen, I. E. M. Kloosterman, G. Pacheco-López, and A. W. M. Evers, "Food Anticipatory Hormonal Responses: A Systematic Review of Animal and Human Studies," *Neuroscience and Biobehavioral Reviews* 126 (2021): 447–464, doi:10.1016/j.neubiorev.2021.03.030.

5. S. Klosterhalfen, A. Rüttgers, E. Krumrey, B. Otto, U. Stockhorst, R. L. Riepl, T. Probst, and P. Enck, "Pavlovian Conditioning of Taste Aversion Using a Motion Sickness Paradigm," *Psychosomatic Medicine* 62, no. 5 (2000): 671–677, doi:10.1097/00006842-200009000-00011.

6. A. van der Meer, N. M. Wulffraat, B. J. Prakken, B. Gijsbers, C. M. Rademaker, and G. Sinnema, "Psychological Side Effects of MTX Treatment in Juvenile Idiopathic Arthritis: A Pilot Study," *Clinical and Experimental Rheumatology* 25, no. 3 (2007): 480–485.

7. F. Benedetti, G. Maggi, L. Lopiano, M. Lanotte, I. Rainero, S. Vighetti, and A. Pollo, "Open Versus Hidden Medical Treatments: The Patient's Knowledge About a Therapy Affects the Therapy Outcome," *Prevention and Treatment* 6, no. 1 (2003): art. 1a, https://doi.org/10.1037/1522-3736.6.1.61a.

8. B. Glintborg, I. J. Sørensen, A. G. Loft, H. Lindegaard, A. Linauskas, O. Hendricks, I. M. Jensen Hansen, et al., "A Nationwide Non-Medical Switch from Originator Infliximab to Biosimilar CT-P13 in 802 Patients with Inflammatory Arthritis: 1-Year Clinical Outcomes from the DANBIO Registry," *Annals of the Rheumatic Diseases* 76, no. 8 (2017): 1426–1431, doi:10.1136/annrheumdis-2016-210742.

9. E. van Overbeeke, B. De Beleyr, J. de Hoon, R. Westhovens, and I. Huys, "Perception of Originator Biologics and Biosimilars: A Survey Among Belgian Rheumatoid Arthritis Patients and Rheumatologists," *BioDrugs* 31, no. 5 (2017): 447–459, doi:10.1007/s40259-017-0244-3.

10. Glintborg et al., "A Nationwide Non-Medical Switch."

11. D. Varelmann, C. Pancaro, E. C. Cappiello, and W. R. Camann, "Nocebo-Induced Hyperalgesia During Local Anesthetic Injection," *Anesthesia and Analg*esia 110, no. 3 (2010): 868–870, doi:10.1213/ANE.0b013e3181cc5727.

12. Varelmann et al., "Nocebo-Induced Hyperalgesia During Local Anesthetic Injection."

13. J. N. Mackenzie, "The Production of the So-Called 'Rose Cold' by Means of an Artificial Rose, with Remarks and Historical Notes," *American Journal of the Medical Sciences* 91, no. 181 (1886): 45.

14. M. Gauci, A. J. Husband, H. Saxarra, and M. G. King, "Pavlovian Conditioning of Nasal Tryptase Release in Human Subjects with Allergic Rhinitis," *Physiology and Behavior* 55, no. 5 (1994): 823–825, doi:10.1016/0031-9384(94)90066-3.

15. R. M. Smits, D. S. Veldhuijzen, H. van Middendorp, M. J. E. van der Heijden, M. van Dijk, and A. W. M. Evers, "Integrating Placebo Effects in General Practice: A Cross-Sectional Survey to Investigate Perspectives from Health Care Professionals in the Netherlands," *Frontiers in Psychiatry* 12 (2021): 768135, doi:10.3389/fpsyt.2021.768135.

CHAPTER 2: WHEN PSYCHOTHERAPY HARMS

1. S. Rosenzweig, "Some Implicit Common Factors in Diverse Methods of Psychotherapy," *American Journal of Orthopsychiatry* 6 (1936): 412–415, https://doi.org/10.1111/j.1939-0025.1936.tb05248.x.

2. C. Locher, S. Meier, and J. Gaab, "Psychotherapy: A World of Meanings," *Frontiers in Psychology* 10 (2019): 460, https://doi.org/10.3389/fpsyg.2019.00460.

3. A. T. Beck, "Beyond Belief: A Theory of Modes, Personality, and Psychopathology," in *Frontiers of Cognitive Psychology*, edited by P. M. Salkovskis, 1–25 (New York: Guilford Press, 1996).

4. B. E. Wampold and Z. E. Imel, *The Great Psychotherapy Debate: The Evidence for What Makes Psychotherapy Work*, 2nd ed. (New York: Routledge, 2015).

5. J. Gaab, C. Blease, C. Locher, and H. Gerger, "Go Open: A Plea for Transparency in Psychotherapy," *Psychology of Consciousness: Theory, Research, and Practice* 3 (2016): 175–198, https://doi.org/10.1037/cns0000063; S. G. Hofmann and S. C. Hayes, "The Future of Intervention Science: Process-Based Therapy," *Clinical Psychological Science* 7 (2019): 37–50, https://doi.org/10.1177/2167702618772296.

6. P. Cuijpers, E. Driessen, S. D. Hollon, P. van Oppen, J. Barth, and G. Andersson, "The Efficacy of Non-Directive Supportive Therapy for Adult Depression: A Meta-Analysis," *Clinical Psychology Review* 32 (2012): 280–291, https://doi.org/10.1016/j.cpr.2012.01.003.

7. M. Greville-Harris and P. Dieppe, "Bad Is More Powerful Than Good: The Nocebo Response in Medical Consultations," *American Journal of Medicine* 128 (2015): 126–129, https://doi.org/10.1016/j.amjmed.2014.08.031.

8. C. Locher, H. Koechlin, J. Gaab, and H. Gerger, "The Other Side of the Coin: Nocebo Effects and Psychotherapy," *Frontiers in Psychiatry* 10 (2019): 555.

9. R. R. Bootzin and E. T. Bailey, "Understanding Placebo, Nocebo, and Iatrogenic Treatment Effects," *Journal of Clinical Psychology* 61 (2005): 871–880, https://doi.org/10.1002/jclp.20131. On non-negative effects, see chapter 4 in this volume, "What Is the Nocebo Effect? A Philosophical Perspective," by Charlotte Blease.

10. T. A. Furukawa, H. Noma, D. M. Caldwell, M. Honyashiki, K. Shinohara, H. Imai, P. Chen, V. Hunot, and R. Churchill, "Waiting List

May Be a Nocebo Condition in Psychotherapy Trials: A Contribution from Network Meta-Analysis," *Acta Psychiatrica Scandinavica* 130 (2014): 181–192, https://doi.org/10.1111/acps.12275.

11. T. W. Baskin, S. C. Tierney, T. Minami, and B. E. Wampold, "Establishing Specificity in Psychotherapy: A Meta-Analysis of Structural Equivalence of Placebo Controls," *Journal of Consulting and Clinical Psychology* 71 (2003): 973.

12. Greville-Harris and Dieppe, "Bad Is More Powerful Than Good."

13. W. Rief, S. G. Hofmann, and Y. Nestoriuc, "The Power of Expectation—Understanding the Placebo and Nocebo Phenomenon," *Social and Personality Psychology Compass* 2 (2008): 1624–1637, https://doi.org/10.1111/j.1751-9004.2008.00121.x.

14. F. Benedetti, M. Lanotte, L. Lopiano, and L. Colloca, "When Words Are Painful: Unraveling the Mechanisms of the Nocebo Effect," *Neuroscience* 147 (2007): 260–271, https://doi.org/10.1016/j.neuroscience.2007.02.020.

15. W. Häuser, E. Hansen, and P. Enck, "Nocebo Phenomena in Medicine: Their Relevance in Everyday Clinical Practice," *Deutsches Ärzteblatt International* 109 (2012): 459–465, https://doi.org/10.3238/arztebl.2012.0459.

16. V. Chavarria, J. Vian, C. Pereira, J. Data-Franco, B. S. Fernandes, M. Berk, and S. Dodd, "The Placebo and Nocebo Phenomena: Their Clinical Management and Impact on Treatment Outcomes," *Clinical Therapeutics* 39 (2017): 477–486, https://doi.org/10.1016/j.clinthera.2017.01.031; L. Colloca and F. G. Miller, "The Nocebo Effect and Its Relevance for Clinical Practice," *Psychosomatic Medicine* 73 (2011): 598–603, https://doi.org/10.1097/PSY.0b013e3182294a50.

17. I. Ladwig, W. Rief, and Y. Nestoriuc, "What Are the Risks and Side Effects of Psychotherapy? Development of an Inventory for the Assessment of Negative Effects of Psychotherapy (INEP)," *Verhaltenstherapie* 24 (2014): 252–263.

18. C. R. Blease, S. O. Lilienfeld, and J. M. Kelley, "Evidence-Based Practice and Psychological Treatments: The Imperatives of Informed Consent," *Frontiers in Psychology* 7 (2016):1170, doi:10.3389/fpsyg.2016.01170.

19. H. Richmond, A. M. Hall, B. Copsey, Z. Hansen, E. Williamson, N. Hoxey-Thomas, Z. Cooper, and S. E. Lamb, "The Effectiveness of Cognitive Behavioural Treatment for Non-Specific Low Back Pain: A Systematic Review and Meta-Analysis," *PLoS One* 10 (2015): e0134192, https://doi.org/10.1371/journal.pone.0134192.

20. N. E. Foster, J. R. Anema, D. Cherkin, R. Chou, S. P. Cohen, D. P. Gross, P. H. Ferreira, et al., "Prevention and Treatment of Low Back Pain: Evidence, Challenges, and Promising Directions," *Lancet* 391 (2018): 2368–2383, https://doi.org/10.1016/S0140-6736(18)30489-6.

21. Locher et al., "The Other Side of the Coin."

22. S. G. Young, C. J. Hayes, J. Aram, and M. A. Tait, "Doctor Hopping and Doctor Shopping for Prescription Opioids Associated with Increased Odds of High-Risk Use," *Pharmacoepidemiology and Drug Safety* 28 (2019): 1117–1124, https://doi.org/10.1002/pds.4838.

23. N. L. Schechter, "Functional Pain: Time for a New Name," *JAMA Pediatrics* 168 (2014): 693–694, https://doi.org/10.1001/jamapediatrics.2014.530.

24. M. E. Hyland, C. Hinton, C. Hill, B. Whalley, R. C. Jones, and A. F. Davies, "Explaining Unexplained Pain to Fibromyalgia Patients: Finding a Narrative That Is Acceptable to Patients and Provides a Rationale for Evidence Based Interventions," *British Journal of Pain* 10 (2016): 156–161, https://doi.org/10.1177/2049463716642601.

25. M. Nicholas, J. W. S. Vlaeyen, W. Rief, A. Barke, Q. Aziz, R. Benoliel, M. Cohen, S. Evers, M. A. Giamberardino, and A. Goebel, "The IASP Classification of Chronic Pain for ICD-11: Chronic Primary Pain," *Pain* 160 (2019): 28–37; R. D. Treede, W. Rief, A. Barke, Q. Aziz, M. I. Bennett, R. Benoliel, M. Cohen, S. Evers, N. B. Finnerup, M. B. First, et al., "Chronic Pain as a Symptom or a Disease: The IASP Classification of Chronic Pain for the International Classification of Diseases (ICD-11)," *Pain* 160 (2019): 19–27, https://doi.org/10.1097/j.pain.0000000000001384.

26. R. Coakley and N. Schechter, "Chronic Pain Is Like . . . : The Clinical Use of Analogy and Metaphor in the Treatment of Chronic Pain in Children," *Pediatric Pain Letter* 15 (2013): 1–8.

27. Hyland et al., "Explaining Unexplained Pain to Fibromyalgia Patients."

CHAPTER 3: THE NOCEBO EFFECT AND COVID-19

1. M. P. S. Yeung, F. L. Y. Yam, and R. Coker, "Factors Associated with the Uptake of Seasonal Influenza Vaccination in Adults: A Systematic Review," *Journal of Public Health* 38, no. 4 (2016): 746–753, doi:10.1093/pubmed/fdv194.

2. S. Taylor, C. A. Landry, M. M. Paluszek, R. Groenewoud, G. S. Rachor, and G. J. G. Asmundson, "A Proactive Approach for Managing COVID-19: The Importance of Understanding the Motivational Roots of Vaccination Hesitancy for SARS-CoV2," *Frontiers in Psychology* 11 (2020): 575950, doi:10.3389/fpsyg.2020.575950.

3. M. Amanzio, D. D. Mitsikostas, F. Giovannelli, M. Bartoli, G. E. Cipriani, and W. A. Brown, "Adverse Events of Active and Placebo Groups in SARS-CoV-2 Vaccine Randomized Trials: A Systematic Review," *Lancet Regional Health—Europe* 12 (2022): 100253, doi:10.1016/j.lanepe.2021.100253; J. W. Haas, F. L. Bender, S. Ballou, J. M. Kelley, M. Wilhelm, F. G. Miller, W. Rief, and T. J. Kaptchuk, "Frequency of Adverse Events in the Placebo Arms of COVID-19 Vaccine Trials: A Systematic Review and Meta-Analysis," *JAMA Network Open* 5, no. 1

(2022): e21423955, doi:10.1001/jamanetworkopen.2021.43955; Y. H. Lee and G. G. Song, "Nocebo Responses in Randomized Controlled Trials of COVID-19 Vaccines," *International Journal of Clinical Pharmacology and Therapeutics* 60, no. 1 (2021): 5–12, doi:10.5414/cp204028.

4. Amanzio et al., "Adverse Events of Active and Placebo Groups."

5. Haas et al., "Frequency of Adverse Events in the Placebo Arms."

6. A. L. Geers, K. S. Clemens, B. Colagiuri, R. Webster, L. Vase, M. Sieg, E. Jason, and L. Colloca, "Psychosocial Factors Predict COVID-19 Vaccine Side Effects," *Psychotherapy and Psychosomatics* 91, no. 2 (2022): 136–138, doi:10.1159/000519853.

7. Y. S. G. Hoffman, Y. Levin, Y. Palgi, R. Goodwin, M. Ben-Ezra, and L. Greenblatt-Kimron, "COVID-19 Vaccine Hesitancy Prospectively Predicts Booster Vaccination Side-Effects Six Months Later: Implications of This Psychosomatic Nocebo Component," 2022, doi:10.21203 /rs.3.rs-1704655/v1.

8. R. K. Webster, J. Weinman, and G. J. Rubin, "Medicine-Related Beliefs Predict Attribution of Symptoms to a Sham Medicine: A Prospective Study," *British Journal of Health Psychology* 23, no. 2 (2018): 436–454, doi:10.1111/bjhp.12298.

9. J. K. Ward, F. Gauna, A. Gagneux-Brunon, E. Botelho-Nevers, J.-L. Cracowski, C. Khouri, O. Launay, P. Verger, and P. Peretti-Watel, "The French Health Pass Holds Lessons for Mandatory COVID-19 Vaccination," *Nature Medicine* 28 (2022): 232–235, doi:10.1038 /s41591-021-01661-7.

10. A. A. Siguan, "Conspiracies and the Nocebo Effect During the COVID-19 Pandemic," *Journal of Public Health* 44, no. 4 (2022): e623–e624, doi:10.1093/pubmed/fdab327.

11. S. Wood and K. Schulman, "Beyond Politics—Promoting Covid-19 Vaccination in the United States," *New England Journal of Medicine* 384 (2021): e23, doi:10.1056/NEJMms2033790.

12. N. Barda, N. Dagan, Y. Ben-Shlomi, E. Kepten, J. Waxman, R. Ohana, M. A. Hernán, et al., "Safety of the BNT162b2 mRNA Covid-19 Vaccine in a Nationwide Setting," *New England Journal of Medicine* 385 (2021): 1078–1090, doi:10.1056/NEJMoa2110475.

13. K. J. Petrie, K. Faasse, F. Crichton, and A. Grey, "How Common Are Symptoms? Evidence from a New Zealand National Telephone Survey," *BMJ Open* 4, no. 6 (2014): e005374, doi:10.1136/ bmjopen-2014-005374.

14. K. MacKrill, "Impact of Media Coverage on Side Effect Reports from the COVID-19 Vaccine," *Journal of Psychosomatic Research* 164 (2023): 111093, doi:10.1016/j.jpsychores.2022.111093.

15. M. Shevlin, E. Nolan, M. Owczarek, O. McBride, J. Murphy, J. Gibson Miller, T. K. Hartman, et al., "COVID-19-Related Anxiety Predicts

Somatic Symptoms in the UK Population," *British Journal of Health Psychology* 25, no. 4 (2020): 875–882, doi:10.1111/bjhp.12430.

16. J. Matta, E. Wiernik, O. Robineau, F. Carrat, M. Touvier, G. Severi, X. de Lamballerie, et al., "Association of Self-Reported COVID-19 Infection and SARS-CoV-2 Serology Test Results with Persistent Physical Symptoms Among French Adults During the COVID-19 Pandemic," *JAMA Internal Medicine* 182, no. 1 (2022): 19–25, doi:10.1001/jamainternmed.2021.6454.

17. H. Daniali and M. A. Flaten, "Experiencing COVID-19 Symptoms Without the Disease: The Role of Nocebo in Reporting of Symptoms," *Scandinavian Journal of Public Health* 50, no. 1 (2022): 61–69, doi:10.1177/14034948211018385.

18. L. Rozenkrantz, T. Kube, M. H. Bernstein, and J. D. E. Gabrieli, "How Beliefs About Coronavirus Disease (COVID) Influence COVID-Like Symptoms?—A Longitudinal Study," *Health Psychology* 41, no. 8 (2022): 519–526, doi:10.1037/HEA0001219.

19. V. van Mulukom, L. J. Pummerer, S. Alper, H. Bai, V. Čavojová, J. Farias, C. S. Kay, et al., "Antecedents and Consequences of COVID-19 Conspiracy Beliefs: A Systematic Review," *Social Science and Medicine* 301 (2022): 114912, doi:10.1016/j.socscimed.2022.114912.

20. L. C. Howe, K. A. Leibowitz, M. A. Perry, J. M. Bitler, W. Block, T. J. Kaptchuk, K. C. Nadeau, and A. J. Crum, "Changing Patient Mindsets About Non-Life-Threatening Symptoms During Oral Immunotherapy: A Randomized Clinical Trial," *Journal of Allergy and Clinical Immunology: In Practice* 7, no. 5 (2019): 1550–1559, doi:10.1016/j.jaip.2019.01.022; W. Rief, "Fear of Adverse Effects and COVID-19 Vaccine Hesitancy: Recommendations of the Treatment Expectation Expert Group," *JAMA Health Forum* 2, no. 4 (2021): e210804, doi:10.1001/jamahealthforum.2021.0804.

21. E. Mahase, "AstraZeneca Vaccine: Blood Clots Are 'Extremely Rare' and Benefits Outweigh Risks, Regulators Conclude," *BMJ* 373 (2021): n931, doi:https://doi.org/10.1136/bmj.n931.

22. M. E. Singer, I. B. Taub, and D. C. Kaelber, "Risk of Myocarditis from COVID-19 Infection in People Under Age 20: A Population-Based Analysis," *MedRxiv*, March 21, 2022, 2021.07.23.21260998, doi:10.1101/2021.07.23.21260998.

CHAPTER 4: WHAT IS THE NOCEBO EFFECT?

1. S. Berry, "The Nocebo Effect: Can Our Thoughts Kill Us?," *Sydney Morning Herald*, March 4, 2015, https://www.smh.com.au/lifestyle/the-nocebo-effect-can-our-thoughts-kill-us-20150303-13tdjl.html.

2. E. Inglis-Arkell, "How the 'Nocebo Effect' Can Trick Us into Actually Dying," Gizmodo, January 26, 2015, https://gizmodo.com /how-the-nocebo-effect-can-trick-us-into-actually-dyin-1681746203.

3. W. B. Cannon, "'Voodoo' Death," *American Anthropologist* 44, no. 2 (1942): 169–181, doi:doi/abs/10.1525/aa.1942.44.2.02a00010.

4. J. Howick and T. Hoffmann, "How Placebo Characteristics Can Influence Estimates of Intervention Effects in Trials," *CMAJ* 190, no. 30 (2018): E908–E911; A. Turner, "'Placebos' and the Logic of Placebo Comparison," *Biology and Philosophy* 27, no. 3 (2012): 419–432.

5. A. Hróbjartsson, T. J. Kaptchuk, and F. G. Miller, "Placebo Effect Studies Are Susceptible to Response Bias and to Other Types of Biases," *Journal of Clinical Epidemiology* 64, no. 11 (2011): 1223–1229; C. Blease, B. Colagiuri, and C. Locher, "Replication Crisis and Placebo Studies: Rebooting the Bioethical Debate," *Journal of Medical Ethics*, published online January 6, 2023, http://dx.doi.org/10.1136/jme-2022-108672; C. G. Maher, A. C. Traeger, C. Abdel Shaheed, and M. O'Keeffe, "Placebos in Clinical Care: A Suggestion Beyond the Evidence," *Medical Journal of Australia* 215, no. 6 (2021): 252–253; C. R. Blease, M. H. Bernstein, and C. Locher, "Open-Label Placebo Clinical Trials: Is It the Rationale, the Interaction or the Pill?," *BMJ Evidence-Based Medicine* 25, no. 5 (2020): 159–165.

6. C. Blease and M. Annoni, "Overcoming Disagreement: A Roadmap for Placebo Studies," *Biology and Philosophy* 34, no. 2 (2019): 18.

7. M. H. Bernstein, C. Locher, S. Stewart-Ferrer, S. Buergler, C. M. DesRoches, M. L. Dossett, F. G. Miller, D. Grose, and C. R. Blease, "Primary Care Providers' Use of and Attitudes Towards Placebos: An Exploratory Focus Group Study with US Physicians," *British Journal of Health Psychology* 25, no. 3 (2020): 596–614, doi:10.1111/bjhp.12429.

8. K. Linde, O. Atmann, K. Meissner, A. Schneider, R. Meister, L. Kriston, and C. Werner, "How Often Do General Practitioners Use Placebos and Non-Specific Interventions? Systematic Review and Meta-Analysis of Surveys," *PLoS One* 13, no. 8 (2018): e0202211, doi:10.1371/journal.pone.0202211.

9. F. Benedetti, *Placebo Effects: Understanding the Mechanisms of Health and Disease* (Oxford: Oxford University Press, 2020).

10. S. Justman, *The Nocebo Effect: Overdiagnosis and Its Costs* (New York: Palgrave Macmillan, 2015).

11. M. Dahl, "How the 'Nocebo Effect' Might Explain Gluten Sensitivity," The Cut, May 28, 2014, https://www.thecut.com/2014/05 /why-so-many-believe-theyre-gluten-sensitive.html.

12. L. Rainie, "E-Patients and Their Hunt for Health Information," Pew Research Center, October 10, 2013, https://www.pewinternet.org/2013/10 /10/e-patients-and-their-hunt-for-health-information/.

13. T. S. Kuhn, *The Structure of Scientific Revolutions* (Chicago: University of Chicago Press, 1962).

14. S. O. Lilienfeld, "Psychology's Replication Crisis and the Grant Culture: Righting the Ship," *Perspectives on Psychological Science* 12, no. 4 (2017): 660–664, doi:10.1177/1745691616687745.

15. D. P. Phillips, G. C. Liu, K. Kwok, J. R. Jarvinen, W. Zhang, and I. S. Abramson, "The *Hound of the Baskervilles* Effect: Natural Experiment on the Influence of Psychological Stress on Timing of Death," *BMJ* 323, no. 7327 (2001): 1443–1446, doi:10.1136/bmj.323.7327.1443.

16. E. M. Sternberg, "Walter B. Cannon and 'Voodoo' Death: A Perspective from 60 Years On," *American Journal of Public Health* 92, no. 10 (2002): 1564–1566, doi:10.2105/ajph.92.10.1564.

CHAPTER 5: THE BIOLOGY OF NOCEBO EFFECTS

1. L. Colloca and A. J. Barsky, "Placebo and Nocebo Effects," *New England Journal of Medicine* 382, no. 6 (2020): 554–561, doi:10.1056/NEJMra1907805.

2. T. J. Luparello, N. Leist, C. H. Lourie, and P. Sweet, "The Interaction of Psychologic Stimuli and Pharmacologic Agents on Airway Reactivity in Asthmatic Subjects," *Psychosomatic Medicine* 32, no. 5 (1970): 509–513, doi:10.1097/00006842-197009000-00009.

3. M. A. Flaten, T. Simonsen, and H. Olsen, "Drug-Related Information Generates Placebo and Nocebo Responses That Modify the Drug Response," *Psychosomatic Medicine* 61, no. 2 (1999): 250–255, doi:10.1097/00006842-199903000-00018.

4. L. Colloca, L. Lopiano, M. Lanotte, and F. Benedetti, "Overt Versus Covert Treatment for Pain, Anxiety, and Parkinson's Disease," *Lancet Neurology* 3, no. 11 (2004): 679–684, doi:10.1016/S1474-4422(04)00908-1.

5. F. Benedetti, L. Colloca, M. Lanotte, B. Bergamasco, E. Torre, and L. Lopiano, "Autonomic and Emotional Responses to Open and Hidden Stimulations of the Human Subthalamic Region," *Brain Research Bulletin* 63, no. 3 (2004): 203–211, doi:10.1016/j.brainresbull.2004.01.010.

6. Colloca et al., "Overt Versus Covert Treatment."

7. Colloca et al., "Overt Versus Covert Treatment."

8. U. Bingel, V. Wanigasekera, K. Wiech, R. Ni Mhuircheartaigh, M. C. Lee, M. Ploner, and I. Tracey, "The Effect of Treatment Expectation on Drug Efficacy: Imaging the Analgesic Benefit of the Opioid Remifentanil," *Science Translational Medicine* 3, no. 70 (2011): 70ra14, doi:10.1126/scitranslmed.3001244.

9. Bingel et al., "The Effect of Treatment Expectation on Drug Efficacy."

10. S. Kessner, K. Wiech, K. Forkmann, M. Ploner, and U. Bingel, "The Effect of Treatment History on Therapeutic Outcome: An Experimental

Approach," *JAMA Internal Medicine* 173, no. 15 (2013): 1468–1469, doi:10.1001/jamainternmed.2013.6705; L. Colloca and F. Benedetti, "How Prior Experience Shapes Placebo Analgesia," *Pain* 124, nos. 1–2 (2006): 126–133, doi:S0304-3959(06)00194-1 [pii] 10.1016/j .pain.2006.04.005.

11. Colloca and Benedetti, "How Prior Experience Shapes Placebo Analgesia."

12. Kessner et al., "The Effect of Treatment History on Therapeutic Outcome."

13. A. Tinnermann, S. Geuter, C. Sprenger, J. Finsterbusch, and C. Buchel, "Interactions Between Brain and Spinal Cord Mediate Value Effects in Nocebo Hyperalgesia," *Science* 358, no. 6359 (2017): 105–108, doi:10.1126/science.aan1221.

14. M. F. van de Sand, M. M. Menz, C. Sprenger, and C. Buchel, "Nocebo-Induced Modulation of Cerebral Itch Processing—An fMRI Study," *NeuroImage* 166 (2018): 209–218, doi:10.1016 /j.neuroimage.2017.10.056.

15. E. Vlemincx, C. Sprenger, and C. Buchel, "Expectation and Dyspnoea: The Neurobiological Basis of Respiratory Nocebo Effects," *European Respiratory Journal* 58, no. 3 (2021): 2003008, doi:10.1183/13993003.03008-2020.

16. Van de Sand et al., "Nocebo-Induced Modulation of Cerebral Itch Processing."

17. F. Benedetti, M. Amanzio, S. Vighetti, and G. Asteggiano, "The Biochemical and Neuroendocrine Bases of the Hyperalgesic Nocebo Effect," *Journal of Neuroscience* 26, no. 46 (2006): 12014–12022, doi:10.1523/JNEUROSCI.2947-06.2006; F. Benedetti, M. Amanzio, C. Casadio, A. Oliaro, and G. Maggi, "Blockade of Nocebo Hyperalgesia by the Cholecystokinin Antagonist Proglumide," *Pain* 71, no. 2 (1997): 135–140, doi:10.1016/s0304-3959(97)03346-0.

18. Benedetti et al., "The Biochemical and Neuroendocrine Bases."

19. J. E. Letzen, T. C. Dildine, C. J. Mun, L. Colloca, S. Bruehl, and C. M. Campbell, "Ethnic Differences in Experimental Pain Responses Following a Paired Verbal Suggestion with Saline Infusion: A Quasiexperimental Study," *Annals of Behavioral Medicine* 55, no. 1 (2021): 55–64, doi:10.1093/abm/kaaa032.

20. R. Shafir, E. Olson, and L. Colloca, "The Neglect of Sex: A Call to Action for Including Sex as a Biological Variable in Placebo and Nocebo Research," *Contemporary Clinical Trials* 116 (2022): 106734, doi:10.1016 /j.cct.2022.106734.

21. E. M. Olson, T. Akintola, J. Phillips, M. Blasini, N. R. Haycock, P. E. Martinez, J. D. Greenspan, S. G. Dorsey, Y. Wang, and L. Colloca, "Effects of Sex on Placebo Effects in Chronic Pain Participants: A Cross-Sectional Study," *Pain* 162, no. 2 (2021): 531–542, doi:10.1097 /j.pain.0000000000002038.

22. P. Enck and S. Klosterhalfen, "Does Sex/Gender Play a Role in Placebo and Nocebo Effects? Conflicting Evidence from Clinical Trials and Experimental Studies," *Frontiers in Neuroscience* 13 (2019): 160, doi:10.3389/fnins.2019.00160.

CHAPTER 6: HOW THE MIND CREATES NOCEBO EFFECTS

1. A. H. Hastorf and H. Cantril, "They Saw a Game: A Case Study," *Journal of Abnormal and Social Psychology* 49, no. 1 (1954): 129–134, doi:10.1037/h0057880.
2. M. von Wernsdorff, M. Loef, B. Tuschen-Caffier, and S. Schmidt, "Effects of Open-Label Placebos in Clinical Trials: A Systematic Review and Meta-Analysis," *Scientific Reports* 11, no. 1 (2021): 3855, doi:10.1038/s41598-021-83148-6.
3. E. B. Titchener, *Experimental Psychology*, 4 vols. (London: Macmillan, 1901).
4. A. J. Barsky and D. A. Silbersweig, "The Amplification of Symptoms in the Medically Ill," *Journal of General Internal Medicine* 38, no. 1 (2022): 195–202, doi:10.1007/s11606-022-07699-8; A. J. Barsky, "The Iatrogenic Potential of the Physician's Words," *Journal of the American Medical Association* 318, no. 24 (2017): 2425–2426, doi:10.1001/jama.2017.16216.
5. M. M. Reidenberg and D. T. Lowenthal, "Adverse Nondrug Reactions," *New England Journal of Medicine* 279, no. 13 (1968): 678–679, doi:10.1056/NEJM196809262791304.
6. R. Collins, C. Reith, J. Emberson, J. Armitage, C. Baigent, L. Blackwell, R. Blumenthal, et al., "Interpretation of the Evidence for the Efficacy and Safety of Statin Therapy," *Lancet* 388, no. 10059 (2016): 2532–2561, doi:10.1016/S0140-6736(16)31357-5.
7. B. A. Ference, H. N. Ginsberg, I. Graham, K. K. Ray, C. J. Packard, E. Bruckert, R. A. Hegele, et al., "Low-Density Lipoproteins Cause Atherosclerotic Cardiovascular Disease. 1. Evidence from Genetic, Epidemiologic, and Clinical Studies. A Consensus Statement from the European Atherosclerosis Society Consensus Panel," *European Heart Journal* 38, no. 32 (2017): 2459–2472, doi:10.1093/eurheartj/ehx144.
8. J. A. Finegold, C. H. Manisty, B. Goldacre, A. J. Barron, and D. P. Francis, "What Proportion of Symptomatic Side Effects in Patients Taking Statins Are Genuinely Caused by the Drug? Systematic Review of Randomized Placebo-Controlled Trials to Aid Individual Patient Choice," *European Journal of Preventive Cardiology* 21, no. 4 (2014): 464–474, doi:10.1177/2047487314525531.
9. F. A. Wood, J. P. Howard, J. A. Finegold, A. N. Nowbar, D. M. Thompson, A. D. Arnold, C. A. Rajkumar, et al., "N-of-1 Trial of a Statin, Placebo, or No Treatment to Assess Side Effects," *New England Journal of Medicine* 383, no. 22 (2020): 2182–2184, doi:10.1056/NEJMc2031173.

10. K. Faasse, G. Gamble, T. Cundy, and K. J. Petrie, "Impact of Television Coverage on the Number and Type of Symptoms Reported During a Health Scare: A Retrospective Pre–Post Observational Study," *BMJ Open* 2, no. 4 (2012): e001607, doi:10.1136/bmjopen-2012-001607.

11. L. C. Howe, K. A. Leibowitz, M. A. Perry, J. M. Bitler, W. Block, T. J. Kaptchuk, K. C. Nadeau, and A. J. Crum, "Changing Patient Mindsets About Non-Life-Threatening Symptoms During Oral Immunotherapy: A Randomized Clinical Trial," *Journal of Allergy and Clinical Immunology: In Practice* 7, no. 5 (2019): 1550–1559, doi:10.1016/j.jaip.2019.01.022.

CHAPTER 7: THE ETHICS OF NOCEBO EFFECTS

1. D. Papadopoulos and D. D. Mitsikostas, "A Meta-Analytic Approach to Estimating Nocebo Effects in Neuropathic Pain Trials," *Journal of Neurology* 259, no. 3 (2012): 436–447, doi:10.1007/s00415-011-6197-4.

2. C. Ma, N. R. Panaccione, T. M. Nguyen, L. Guizzetti, C. E. Parker, I. M. Hussein, N. Vande Casteele, et al., "Adverse Events and Nocebo Effects in Inflammatory Bowel Disease: A Systematic Review and Meta-Analysis of Randomized Controlled Trials," *Journal of Crohn's and Colitis* 13, no. 9 (2019): 1201–1216, doi:10.1093/ecco-jcc/jjz087.

3. D. D. Mitsikostas, L. I. Mantonakis, and N. G. Chalarakis, "Nocebo Is the Enemy, Not Placebo: A Meta-Analysis of Reported Side Effects After Placebo Treatment in Headaches," *Cephalalgia* 31, no. 5 (2011): 550–561, doi:10.1177/0333102410391485.

4. N. Mondaini, P. Gontero, G. Giubilei, G. Lombardi, T. Cai, A. Gavazzi, and R. Bartoletti, "Finasteride 5 mg and Sexual Side Effects: How Many of These Are Related to a Nocebo Phenomenon?," *Journal of Sexual Medicine* 4, no. 6 (2007): 1708–1712, doi:10.1111/j.1743-6109.2007.00563.x.

5. M. Annoni and C. Blease, "Persons over Models: Shared Decision-Making for Person-Centered Medicine," *European Journal for Person Centered Healthcare* 8, no. 3 (2020): 355–362.

6. M. Annoni, "Better Than Nothing: A Historical Account of Placebos and Placebo Effects from Modern to Contemporary Medicine," *International Review of Neurobiology* 153 (2020): 3–26, https://doi.org/10.1016/bs.irn.2020.03.028.

7. A. Surbone, "Truth Telling to the Patient," *Journal of the American Medical Association* 7, no. 268 (1992): 1661–1663.

8. S. J. Baumrucker, M. Stolick, P. Mingle, G. Vandekieft, G. M. Morris, D. Harrington, and K. A. Oertli, "Placebo: Medicine or Deception?," *American Journal of Hospice and Palliative Medicine* 28 (2011): 284–289, doi:10.1177/1049909111402635.

9. Z. Zhang and X. Min, "The Ethical Dilemma of Truth-Telling in Healthcare in China," *Bioethical Inquiry* 17 (2020: 337–344, https://doi.org/10.1007/s11673-020-09979-6.

10. L. Colloca and F. G. Miller, "The Nocebo Effect and Its Relevance for Clinical Practice," *Psychosomatic Medicine* 73, no. 7 (2011): 598–603, doi:10.1097/PSY.0b013e3182294a50.

11. M. Hägglund, C. DesRoches, C. Petersen, and I. Scandurra, "Patients' Access to Health Records," *BMJ* 367 (2019): l5725, https://doi.org/10.1136/bmj.l5725.

12. C. R. Blease, T. Delbanco, J. Torous, M. Ponten, C. M. DesRoches, M. Hägglund, and I. Kirsch, "Sharing Clinical Notes, and Placebo and Nocebo Effects: Can Documentation Affect Patient Health?," *Journal of Health Psychology* 27, no. 1 (2022): 135–146, https://doi.org/10.1177/1359105320948588.

13. J. Walker, S. Leveille, S. Bell, H. Chimowitz, Z. Dong, J. G. Elmore, L. Fernandez, et al., "OpenNotes After 7 Years: Patient Experiences with Ongoing Access to Their Clinicians' Outpatient Visit Notes," *Journal of Medical Internet Research* 21, no. 5 (2019): e13876, doi:10.2196/13876.

14. C. R. Blease, "Sharing Online Clinical Notes with Patients: Implications for Nocebo Effects and Health Equity," *Journal of Medical Ethics*, 49, no. 1 (2023): 14–21, doi:10.1136/jme-2022-108413.

15. C. M. DesRoches, S. K. Bell, Z. Dong, J. Elmore, L. Fernandez, P. Fitzgerald, J. M. Liao, T. H. Payne, T. Delbanco, and J. Walker, "Patients Managing Medications and Reading Their Visit Notes: A Survey of OpenNotes Participants," *Annals of Internal Medicine* 171, no. 1 (2019): 69–71, doi:10.7326/M18-3197.

16. L. Fernández, A. Fossa, Z. Dong, T. Delbanco, J. Elmore, P. Fitzgerald, K. Harcourt, J. Perez, J. Walker, and C. DesRoches, "Words Matter: What Do Patients Find Judgmental or Offensive in Outpatient Notes?," *Journal of General Internal Medicine* 36, no. 9 (2021) 2571–2578, doi:10.1007/s11606-020-06432-7.

17. G. Himmelstein, D. Bates, and L. Zhou, "Examination of Stigmatizing Language in the Electronic Health Record," *JAMA Network Open* 5, no. 1 (2022): e2144967, doi:10.1001/jamanetworkopen.2021.44967.

18. J. Birkhäuer, J. Gaab, J. Kossowsky, S. Hasler, P. Krummenacher, C. Werner, and H. Gerger, "Trust in the Health Care Professional and Health Outcome: A Meta-Analysis," *PLoS One* 12, no. 2 (2017): e0170988, doi:10.1371/journal.pone.0170988.

19. A. J. Barsky, R. Saintfort, M. P. Rogers, and J. F. Borus, "Nonspecific Medication Side Effects and the Nocebo Phenomenon," *Journal of the American Medical Association* 287, no. 5 (2002): 622–627, doi:10.1001/jama.287.5.622.

CHAPTER 8: HOW CLINICIANS CAN
MINIMIZE NOCEBO EFFECTS

1. A. W. M. Evers, L. Colloca, C. Blease, M. Annoni, L. Y. Atlas, F. Benedetti, U. Bingel, et al., "Implications of Placebo and Nocebo Effects for Clinical Practice: Expert Consensus," *Psychotherapy and Psychosomatics* 87, no. 4 (2018): 204–210, doi:10.1159/000490354.

2. R. K. Webster and G. J. Rubin, "Influencing Side-Effects to Medicinal Treatments: A Systematic Review of Brief Psychological Interventions," *Frontiers in Psychiatry* 9 (2019): 775, doi:10.3389/fpsyt.2018.00775.

3. N. Mondaini, P. Gontero, G. Giubilei, G. Lombardi, T. Cai, A. Gavazzi, and R. Bartoletti, "Finasteride 5 mg and Sexual Side Effects: How Many of These Are Related to a Nocebo Phenomenon?," *Journal of Sexual Medicine* 4, no. 6 (2007): 1708–1712, doi:10.1111/j.1743-6109.2007.00563.x.

4. M. Sieg and L. Vase, "Patient Attitudes Towards Side Effect Information: An Important Foundation for the Ethical Discussion of the Nocebo Effect of Informed Consent," *Clinical Ethics*, published online 2022, https://doi.org/10.1177/14777509221077390.

5. F. G. Miller and L. Colloca, "The Placebo Phenomenon and Medical Ethics: Rethinking the Relationship Between Informed Consent and Risk-Benefit Assessment," *Theoretical Medicine and Bioethics* 32, no. 4 (2011): 229–243, doi:10.1007/s11017-011-9179-8.

6. M. Alfano, "Placebo Effects and Informed Consent," *American Journal of Bioethics* 15, no. 10 (2015): 3–12, https://doi.org/10.1080/15265161.2015.1074302.

7. Alfano, "Placebo Effects and Informed Consent."

8. C. Blease, "Authorized Concealment and Authorized Deception: Well-Intended Secrets Are Likely to Induce Nocebo Effects," *American Journal of Bioethics* 15, no. 10 (2015): 23–25, https://doi.org/10.1080/15265161.2015.1074310.

9. K. Barnes, K. Faasse, A. L. Geers, S. G. Helfer, L. Sharpe, L. Colloca, and B. Colagiuri, "Can Positive Framing Reduce Nocebo Side Effects? Current Evidence and Recommendation for Future Research," *Frontiers in Pharmacology* 10 (2019): 167, doi:10.3389/fphar.2019.00167.

10. A. Mao, K. Barnes, L. Sharpe, A. L. Geers, S. G. Helfer, K. Faasse, and B. Colagiuri, "Using Positive Attribute Framing to Attenuate Nocebo Side Effects: A Cybersickness Study," *Annals of Behavioral Medicine* 55, no. 8 (2021): 769–778, doi:10.1093/abm/kaaa115.

11. S. G. Helfer, B. Colagiuri, K. Faasse, K. S. Clemens, F. Caplandies, and A. L. Geers, "The Influence of Message Framing on Nocebo Headaches: Findings from a Randomized Laboratory Design," *Journal of Behavioral Medicine* 45, no. 3 (2022): 438–450, doi:10.1007/s10865-022-00294-6.

12. Barnes et al., "Can Positive Framing Reduce Nocebo Side Effects?"

13. E. Peters, P. S. Hart, and L. Fraenkel, "Informing Patients: The Influence of Numeracy, Framing, and Format of Side Effect Information on Risk Perceptions," *Medical Decision Making* 31, no. 3 (2011): 432–436, doi:10.1177/0272989X10391672.

14. R. K. Webster and G. J. Rubin, "Predicting Expectations of Side-Effects for Those Which Are Warned Versus Not Warned About in Patient Information Leaflets," *Annals of Behavioral Medicine* 55, no. 12 (2021): 1253–1261, doi:10.1093/abm/kaab015.

15. T. Kube, J. A. Glombiewski, and W. Rief, "Using Different Expectation Mechanisms to Optimize Treatment of Patients with Medical Conditions: A Systematic Review," *Psychosomatic Medicine* 80, no. 6 (2018): 535–543, doi:10.1097/PSY.0000000000000596.

16. Y. Pan, T. Kinitz, M. Stapic, and Y. Nestoriuc, "Minimizing Drug Adverse Events by Informing About the Nocebo Effect—An Experimental Study," *Frontiers in Psychiatry* 10 (2019): 504, doi:10.3389/fpsyt.2019.00504.

17. T. Michnevich, Y. Pan, A. Hendi, K. Oechsle, A. Stein, and Y. Nestoriuc, "Preventing Adverse Events of Chemotherapy for Gastrointestinal Cancer by Educating Patients About the Nocebo Effect: A Randomized-Controlled Trial," *BMC Cancer* 22, no. 1 (2022): 1008, doi:10.1186/s12885-022-10089-2.

18. Y. Nestoriuc, Y. Pan, T. Kinitz, E. Weik, and M. C. Shedden-Mora, "Informing About the Nocebo Effect Affects Patients' Need for Information About Antidepressants—An Experimental Online Study," *Frontiers in Psychiatry* 12 (2021): 587233, doi:10.3389/fpsyt.2021.587122.

19. A. L. Geers, K. Faasse, D. A. Guevarra, K. S. Clemens, S. G. Helfer, and B. Colagiuri, "Affect and Emotions in Placebo and Nocebo Effects: What Do We Know So Far?," *Social and Personality Psychology Compass* 15, no. 1 (2021): e12575, https://doi.org/10.1111/spc3.12575.

20. A. L. Geers, S. Close, F. C. Caplandies, and L. Vase, "A Positive Mood Induction for Reducing the Formation of Nocebo Effects from Side Effect Information," *Annals of Behavioral Medicine* 53, no. 11 (2019): 999–1008, doi:10.1093/abm/kaz005.

21. L. C. Howe, J. P. Goyer, and A. J. Crum, "Harnessing the Placebo Effect: Exploring the Influence of Physician Characteristics on Placebo Response," *Health Psychology* 36, no. 11 (2017): 1074–1082, doi:10.1037/hea0001235.

22. J. M. Kelley, G. Kraft-Todd, L. Schapira, J. Kossowsky, and H. Riess, "The Influence of the Patient-Clinician Relationship on Healthcare Outcomes: A Systematic Review and Meta-Analysis of Randomized Controlled Trials," *PLoS One* 9, no. 4 (2014): e94207, doi:10.1371/journal.pone.0094207.

23. M. Greville-Harris and P. Dieppe, "Bad Is More Powerful Than Good: The Nocebo Response in Medical Consultations," *American Journal of Medicine* 128, no. 2 (2015): 126–129, doi:10.1016/j.amjmed.2014.08.031.

24. R. H. Gracely, R. Dubner, W. R. Deeter, and P. J. Wolskee, "Clinicians' Expectations Influence Placebo Analgesia," *Lancet* 1, no. 8419 (1985): 43, doi:10.1016/s0140-6736(85)90984-5.

25. D. Varelmann, C. Pancaro, E. C. Cappiello, and W. R. Camann, "Nocebo-Induced Hyperalgesia During Local Anesthetic Injection," *Anesthesia and Analgesia* 110, no. 3 (2010): 868–870, doi:10.1213/ANE.0b013e3181cc5727.

26. U. Bingel, V. Wanigasekera, K. Wiech, R. Ni Mhuircheartaigh, M. C. Lee, M. Ploner, and I. Tracey, "The Effect of Treatment Expectation on Drug Efficacy: Imaging the Analgesic Benefit of the Opioid Remifentanil," *Science Translational Medicine* 3, no. 70 (2011): 70ra14, doi:10.1126/scitranslmed.3001244.

CHAPTER 9: PROTECTING YOURSELF FROM NOCEBO EFFECTS

1. S. Cohen, "The Nocebo Effect of Informed Consent," *Bioethics* 28, no. 3 (2014): 147–154, doi:10.1111/j.1467-8519.2012.01983.x.

2. M. Alfano, "Placebo Effects and Informed Consent," *American Journal of Bioethics* 15, no. 10 (2015): 3–12, https://doi.org/10.1080/15265161.2015.1074302.

3. A. Weil, *Spontaneous Healing* (New York: Knopf, 1995).

CHAPTER 10: NOCEBO, THE ENVIRONMENT, AND PUBLIC HEALTH

1. T. F. Jones, A. S. Craig, D. Hoy, E. Gunter, D. L. Ashley, D. B. Barr, J. W. Brock, and W. Schaffner, "Mass Psychogenic Illness Attributed to Toxic Exposure at a High School," *New England Journal of Medicine* 342, no. 2 (2000): 96–100, doi:10.1056/NEJM200001133420206.

2. C. Baliatsas, I. Van Kamp, E. Lebret, and G. J. Rubin, "Idiopathic Environmental Intolerance Attributed to Electromagnetic Fields (IEI-EMF): A Systematic Review of Identifying Criteria," *BMC Public Health* 12, no. 1 (2012): 1–23, doi:10.1186/1471-2458-12-643.

3. TNS Opinion and Social, "Electromagnetic Fields," Special Eurobarometer 347 / Wave 73.3, European Commission, Brussels, June 2010, https://europa.eu/eurobarometer/surveys/detail/843.

4. M. Feychting, A. Ahlbom, and L. Kheifets, "EMF and Health," *Annual Review of Public Health* 26, no. 1 (2005): 165–189, doi:10.1146/annurev.publhealth.26.021304.144445.

5. A. Ahlbom, N. Day, M. Feychting, E. Roman, J. Skinner, J. Dockerty, M. Linet, et al., "A Pooled Analysis of Magnetic Fields and Childhood Leukaemia," *British Journal of Cancer* 83, no. 5 (2000): 692–698, doi:10.1054/bjoc.2000.1376.

6. M. Repacholi, "Concern That 'EMF' Magnetic Fields from Power Lines Cause Cancer," *Science of the Total Environment* 426 (2012): 454–458, doi:10.1016/j.scitotenv.2012.03.030.

7. World Health Organization, *Extremely Low Frequency Fields*, Environmental Health Criteria Monograph No. 238 (Geneva: WHO, 2007), https://www.who.int/publications/i/item/9789241572385.

8. K. J. Petrie, E. A. Broadbent, N. Kley, R. Moss-Morris, R. Horne, and W. Rief, "Worries About Modernity Predict Symptom Complaints After Environmental Pesticide Spraying," *Psychosomatic Medicine* 67, no. 5 (2005): 778–782, doi:10.1097/01.psy.0000181277.48575.a4.

9. E. Palmquist, K. J. Petrie, and S. Nordin, "Psychometric Properties and Normative Data for a Swedish Version of the Modern Health Worries Scale," *International Journal of Behavioral Medicine* 24, no. 1 (2017): 54–65, doi:10.1007/s12529-016-9576-5.

10. P. Slovic, "Perception of Risk," *Science* 236, no. 4799 (1987): 280–285, doi:10.1126/science.3563507.

11. M. G. Morgan, P. Slovic, I. Nair, D. Geisler, D. MacGregor, B. Fischhoff, D. Lincoln, and K. Florig, "Powerline Frequency Electric and Magnetic Fields: A Pilot Study of Risk Perception," *Risk Analysis* 5, no. 2 (1985): 139–149, doi:10.1111/j.1539-6924.1985.tb00161.x.

12. R. Szemerszky, F. Köteles, R. Lihi, and G. Bárdos, "Polluted Places or Polluted Minds? An Experimental Sham-Exposure Study on Background Psychological Factors of Symptom Formation in 'Idiophatic [*sic*] Environmental Intolerance Attributed to Electromagnetic Fields,'" *International Journal of Hygiene and Environmental Health* 213, no. 5 (2010): 387–394, https://doi.org/10.1016/j.ijheh.2010.05.001.

13. M. Witthöft and G. J. Rubin, "Are Media Warnings About the Adverse Health Effects of Modern Life Self-Fulfilling? An Experimental Study on Idiopathic Environmental Intolerance Attributed to Electromagnetic Fields (IEI-EMF)," *Journal of Psychosomatic Research* 74, no. 3 (2013): 206–212, doi:10.1016/j.jpsychores.2012.12.002.

14. F. Crichton, G. Dodd, G. Schmid, G. Gamble, and K. J. Petrie, "Can Expectations Produce Symptoms from Infrasound Associated with Wind Turbines?," *Health Psychology* 33, no. 4 (2014): 360, doi:10.1037/a0031760.

15. J. T. Porsius, L. Claassen, T. Smid, F. Woudenberg, and D. R. M. Timmermans, "Health Responses to a New High-Voltage Power Line Route: Design of a Quasi-Experimental Prospective Field Study in the Netherlands," *BMC Public Health* 14, no. 1 (2014): 1–12, doi:10.1186/1471-2458-14-237.

16. J. T. Porsius, L. Claassen, T. Smid, F. Woudenberg, K. J. Petrie, and D. R. M. Timmermans, "Symptom Reporting After the Introduction of a New High-Voltage Power Line: A Prospective Field Study," *Environmental Research* 138 (2015): 112–117, doi:10.1016/j.envres.2015.02.009.

17. World Health Organization, *Extremely Low Frequency Fields*.
18. G. J. Rubin, R. Nieto-Hernandez, and S. Wessely, "Idiopathic Environmental Intolerance Attributed to Electromagnetic Fields (Formerly 'Electromagnetic Hypersensitivity'): An Updated Systematic Review of Provocation Studies," *Bioelectromagnetics* 31, no. 1 (2010): 1–11, doi:10.1002/bem.20536.
19. J. T. Porsius, L. Claassen, F. Woudenberg, T. Smid, and D. R. M. Timmermans, "Nocebo Responses to High-Voltage Power Lines: Evidence from a Prospective Field Study," *Science of the Total Environment* 543 (2016): 432–438, doi:10.1016/j.scitotenv.2015.11.038.
20. J. T. Porsius, L. Claassen, F. Woudenberg, T. Smid, and D. R. M. Timmermans, "'These Power Lines Make Me Ill': A Typology of Residents' Health Responses to a New High-Voltage Power Line," *Risk Analysis* 37, no. 12 (2017): 2276–2288, doi:10.1111/risa.12786.
21. L. Claassen, T. Smid, F. Woudenberg, and D. R. M. Timmermans, "Media Coverage on Electromagnetic Fields and Health: Content Analysis of Dutch Newspaper Articles and Websites," *Health, Risk and Society* 14, nos. 7–8 (2012): 681–696, https://doi.org/10.1080/13698575.2012.716820.
22. J. T. Porsius, L. Claassen, P. E. Weijland, and D. R. M. Timmermans, "'They Give You Lots of Information, but Ignore What It's Really About': Residents' Experiences with the Planned Introduction of a New High-Voltage Power Line," *Journal of Environmental Planning and Management* 59, no. 8 (2016): 1495–1512, https://doi.org/10.1080/09640568.2015.1080672.
23. Porsius et al., "'They Give You Lots of Information.'"
24. Porsius et al., "'They Give You Lots of Information.'"
25. L. A. Page, K. J. Petrie, and S. C. Wessely, "Psychosocial Responses to Environmental Incidents: A Review and a Proposed Typology," *Journal of Psychosomatic Research* 60, no. 4 (2006): 413–422, doi:10.1016/j.jpsychores.2005.11.008.
26. F. Crichton and K. J. Petrie, "Health Complaints and Wind Turbines: The Efficacy of Explaining the Nocebo Response to Reduce Symptom Reporting," *Environmental Research* 140 (2015): 449–455, doi:10.1016/j.envres.2015.04.016.

CHAPTER 11: THE NOCEBO EFFECT AND THE MEDIA

1. Z. Babar, J. Stewart, S. Reddy, W. Alzaher, P. Vareed, N. Yacoub, B. Dhroptee, and A. Rew, "An Evaluation of Consumers' Knowledge, Perceptions and Attitudes Regarding Generic Medicines in Auckland," *Pharmacy World and Science* 32, no. 4 (2010): 440–448, doi:10.1007/s11096-010-9402-0.
2. F. van Hunsel, A. Passier, and K. van Grootheest, "Comparing Patients' and Healthcare Professionals' ADR Reports After Media Attention: The Broadcast of a Dutch Television Programme About the Benefits and Risks

of Statins as an Example," *British Journal of Clinical Pharmacology* 67, no. 5 (2009): 558–564, doi:10.1111/j.1365-2125.2009.03400.x.

3. R. B. Goldszmidt, A. Buttendorf, G. Schuldt Filho, J. M. Souza Jr., and M. A. Bianchini, "The Impact of Generic Labels on the Consumption of and Adherence to Medication: A Randomized Controlled Trial," *European Journal of Public Health* 29, no. 1 (2019): 12–17, doi:10.1093/eurpub/cky183.

4. K. Faasse, T. Cundy, G. Gamble, and K. J. Petrie, "The Effect of an Apparent Change to a Branded or Generic Medication on Drug Effectiveness and Side Effects," *Psychosomatic Medicine* 75, no. 1 (2013): 90–96, doi:10.1097/PSY.0b013e3182738826; P. Blier, H. C. Margolese, E. A. Wilson, and M. Boucher, "Switching Medication Products During the Treatment of Psychiatric Illness," *International Journal of Psychiatry in Clinical Practice* 23, no. 1 (2019): 2–13, doi:10.1080/13651501.2018.1508724.

5. K. MacKrill, G. D. Gamble, D. J. Bean, T. Cundy, and K. J. Petrie, "Evidence of a Media-Induced Nocebo Response Following a Nationwide Antidepressant Drug Switch," *Clinical Psychology in Europe* 1, no. 1 (2019): 1–12, doi:10.32872/cpe.v1i1.29642.

6. P. W. O'Carroll and L. B. Potter, "Suicide Contagion and the Reporting of Suicide: Recommendations from a National Workshop," *Morbidity and Mortality Weekly Report: Recommendations and Reports* 43, RR-6 (1994): 9–18.

7. K. MacKrill, G. D. Gamble, and K. J. Petrie, "The Effect of Television and Print News Stories on the Nocebo Responding Following a Generic Medication Switch," *Clinical Psychology in Europe* 2, no. 2 (2020): e2623, doi:10.32872/cpe.v2i2.2623.

8. M. G. Lauridsen and S. K. Sporrong, "How Does Media Coverage Effect the Consumption of Antidepressants? A Study of the Media Coverage of Antidepressants in Danish Online Newspapers 2010–2011," *Research in Social and Administrative Pharmacy* 14, no. 7 (2018): 638–644, doi:10.1016/j.sapharm.2017.07.011.

9. K. Faasse, J. T. Porsius, J. Faasse, and L. R. Martin, "Bad News: The Influence of News Coverage and Google Searches on Gardasil Adverse Event Reporting," *Vaccine* 35, no. 49, pt. B (2017): 6872–6878, doi:10.1016/j.vaccine.2017.10.004.

10. K. Faasse, G. Gamble, T. Cundy, and K. J. Petrie, "Impact of Television Coverage on the Number and Type of Symptoms Reported During a Health Scare: A Retrospective Pre–Post Observational Study," *BMJ Open* 2, no. 4 (2012): e001607, doi:10.1136/bmjopen-2012-001607.

11. S. Splendore and M. Brambilla, "The Hybrid Journalism That We Do Not Recognize (Anymore)," *Journalism and Media* 2, no. 1 (2021): 51–61, doi:10.3390/journalmedia2010004.

12. "The Potentially Life Threatening Side Effects of Taking Statins," *Daily Express*, February 4, 2021, https://www.express.co.uk/life-style /health/1393571/statins-side-effects-liver-failure-high-cholesterol-alternative.

13. I. P. Hargreaves, J. Lewis, T. Speers, and E. L. Hargreaves, "Towards a Better Map: Science, the Public and the Media," Economic and Social Research Council, 2003.

14. Lauridsen and Sporrong, "How Does Media Coverage Effect the Consumption of Antidepressants?"

15. K. Faasse, A. Grey, R. Jordan, S. Garland, and K. J. Petrie, "Seeing Is Believing: Impact of Social Modeling on Placebo and Nocebo Responding," *Health Psychology* 34, no. 8 (2015): 880–885, doi:10.1037/ hea0000199; E. Vögtle, A. Barke, and B. Kröner-Herwig, "Nocebo Hyperalgesia Induced by Social Observational Learning," *Pain* 154, no. 8 (2013): 1427–1423, doi:10.1016/j.pain.2013.04.041.

16. K. MacKrill, Z. Morrison, and K. J. Petrie, "Increasing and Dampening the Nocebo Response Following Medicine-Taking: A Randomised Controlled Trial," *Journal of Psychosomatic Research* 150 (2021): 110630, doi:10.1016/j.jpsychores.2021.110630.

17. Van Hunsel, Passier, and van Grootheest, "Comparing Patients' and Healthcare Professionals' ADR Reports After Media Attention."

18. S. F. Nielsen and B. G. Nordestgaard, "Negative Statin-Related News Stories Decrease Statin Persistence and Increase Myocardial Infarction and Cardiovascular Mortality: A Nationwide Prospective Cohort Study," *European Heart Journal* 37, no. 11 (2016): 908–916, doi:10.1093/eurheartj /ehv641.

CHAPTER 12: FROM GENITAL-SHRINKING PANICS TO HUMMING GIRAFFES

1. Various media reports cited in R. E. Bartholomew and B. Rickard, *Mass Hysteria in Schools: A Worldwide History Since 1566* (Jefferson, NC: McFarland, 2014).

2. K. Wattanagun, *The Ravenous Spirit (Phii Pob) Belief Permission in Contemporary Thailand: Plural Practices Versus Monolithic Representations*, Ph.D. dissertation, Department of Folklore and Ethnomusicology, Indiana University, 2016.

3. W. I. Thomas, *The Unadjusted Girl: With Cases and Standpoint for Behavior Analysis* (Boston: Little, Brown, 1923).

4. M. Zaragoza, R. F. Belli, and K. E. Payment, "Misinformation Effects and the Suggestibility of Eyewitness Memory," in *Do Justice and Let the Sky Fall: Elizabeth Loftus and Her Contributions to Science, Law, and Academic Freedom*, edited by M. Garry and H. Hayne, 35–64 (Mahwah, NJ: Lawrence Erlbaum, 2007), doi:10.4324/9780203774861-4.

5. "DNA Exonerations in the United States (1989–2020)," Innocence Project, https://innocenceproject.org/dna-exonerations-in-the-united-states/.

6. D. Daegling, *Bigfoot Exposed: An Anthropologist Examines America's Enduring Legend* (Walnut Creek, CA: AltaMira Press, 2004); B. Radford, *Tracking the Chupacabra: The Vampire Beast in Fact, Fiction, and Folklore* (Albuquerque: University of New Mexico Press, 2011).

7. H. Fraser, "The Reliability of Voice Recognition by 'Ear Witnesses': An Overview of Research Findings," *Language and Law/Linguagem e Direito* 6, no. 2 (2019): 1–9, doi:10.21747/21833745/lanlaw/6_2a1.

8. E. McClelland, "Voice Recognition Within a Closed Set of Family Members," paper presented at the International Association for Forensic Phonetics and Acoustics Conference, Swiss Federal Institute of Technology, Lausanne, 2008; L. Öhman, "All Ears: Adults' and Children's Earwitness Testimony," Department of Psychology, University of Gothenburg, 2013, iii.

9. P. Berger and T. Luckmann, *The Social Construction of Reality: A Treatise in the Sociology of Knowledge* (New York: Anchor Books, 1967).

10. J. W. Conner, "Social and Psychological Reality of European Witchcraft Beliefs," *Psychiatry* 38, no. 4 (1975): 366–380.

11. G. A. Leng, "Koro—Its Origin and Nature as a Disease Entity," *Singapore Medical Journal* 9, no. 1 (1968): 3–6.

12. W. S. Tseng, K. M. Mo, J. Hsu, L. S. Li, L. W. Ou, G. Q. Chen, and D. W. Jiang, "A Sociocultural Study of Koro Epidemics in Guangdong, China," *American Journal of Psychiatry* 145, no. 12 (1988): 1538–1543, doi:10.1176/ajp.145.12.1538.

13. R. E. Bartholomew, "The Medicalization of Exotic Deviance: A Sociological Perspective on Epidemic Koro," *Transcultural Psychiatry* 35, no. 1 (1998): 5–38, https://doi.org/10.1177/136346159803500101.

14. Tseng et al., "A Sociocultural Study of Koro Epidemics," 1538.

15. Tseng et al., "A Sociocultural Study of Koro Epidemics," 1540.

16. W. G. Jilek, "Epidemics of 'Genital Shrinking' (Koro): Historical Review and Report of a Recent Outbreak in Southern China," *Curare* 9, nos. 3–4 (1986): 269–282.

17. W. S. Tseng, K. M. Mo, J. Hsu, L. S. Li, L. W. Ou, G. Q. Chen, and D. W. Jiang, "A Socio-Cultural and Clinical Study of a Koro (Genital Retraction Panic Disorder) Epidemic in Guangdong, China," paper presented at the Conference of the Society for the Study of Psychiatry and Culture, Quebec City, Canada, September 16–19, 1987; Tseng et al., "A Sociocultural Study of Koro Epidemics," 1538.

18. W. S. Tseng, K. M. Mo, L. S. Li, G. Q. Chen, L. W. Ou, and H. B. Zheng, "Koro Epidemics in Guangdong, China: A Questionnaire Survey," *Journal of Nervous and Mental Disease* 180, no. 2 (1992): 117–123.

19. Tseng et al., "Koro Epidemics in Guangdong, China," 117; Jilek, "Epidemics of 'Genital Shrinking' (Koro)," 274; H. B. Murphy, "The Koro Epidemic in Hainan Island," paper presented at the Regional Conference of the World Psychiatric Association's Transcultural Psychiatry Section, Beijing, China, August 17–31, 1986.
20. Leng, "Koro—Its Origin and Nature as a Disease Entity."
21. Tseng et al., "A Sociocultural Study of Koro Epidemics."
22. R. W. Baloh and R. E. Bartholomew, *Havana Syndrome: Mass Psychogenic Illness and the Real Story Behind the Embassy Mystery and Hysteria* (Cham, Switzerland: Copernicus Books, 2020).
23. Baloh and Bartholomew, *Havana Syndrome*, 38.
24. Mitre Corporation, "Acoustic Signals and Physiological Effects on U.S. Diplomats in Cuba," study conducted for the U.S. State Department, 2018; R. Bartholomew, "NAS Report on 'Havana Syndrome' Mired in Controversy," *Skeptical Inquirer* 45, no. 2 (2021): 7–8.
25. R. L. Swanson II, S. Hampton, J. Green-McKenzie, R. Diaz-Arrastia, M. S. Grady, R. Verma, R. Biester, D. Duda, R. Wolf, and D. H. Smith, "Neurological Manifestations Among US Government Personnel Reporting Directional Audible and Sensory Phenomena in Havana, Cuba," *Journal of the American Medical Association* 319, no. 11 (2018): 1125–1133, doi:10.1001/jama.2018.1742.
26. R. Verma, R. L. Swanson II, D. Parker, A. A. Ould Ismail, R. T. Shinohara, J. A. Alappatt, J. Doshi, et al., "Neuroimaging Findings in US Government Personnel with Possible Exposure to Directional Phenomena in Havana, Cuba," *Journal of the American Medical Association* 322, no. 4 (2019): 336–347, doi:10.1001/jama.2019.9269.
27. L. Austin, "Anomalous Health Incident. Memorandum for All Department of Defense Employees," U.S. Department of Defense, September 15, 2021.
28. R. E. Bartholomew, "*60 Minutes* Whips Up 'Havana Syndrome' Hysteria, Airing Sensational Segment on White House 'Attacks,'" *Skeptic* 27, no. 2 (2022): 32–36.
29. S. Harris and M. Ryan, "CIA Finds No 'Worldwide Campaign' by Any Foreign Power Behind Mysterious 'Havana Syndrome,'" *Washington Post*, January 20, 2022.
30. J. Kennaway, *Bad Vibrations: The History of the Idea of Music as a Cause of Disease* (London: Taylor & Francis, 2016).
31. J. Kennaway, "Historical Perspectives on Music as a Cause of Disease," in *Music, Neurology, and Neuroscience: Historical Connections and Perspectives,* edited by E. Altenmüller, S. Finger, and F. Boller, Progress in Brain Research, vol. 216, 127–147 (Amsterdam: Elsevier, 2015).
32. S. Finger, *Doctor Stanley's Medicine* (Philadelphia: University of Pennsylvania Press, 2006); D. A. Gallo and S. Finger, "The Power

of a Musical Instrument: Franklin, the Mozarts, Mesmer, and the Glass Armonica," *History of Psychology* 3, no. 4 (2000): 326–343, doi:10.1037/1093-4510.3.4.326.

33. Z. J. Lipowski, "Benjamin Franklin as a Psychotherapist: A Forerunner of Brief Psychotherapy," *Perspectives in Biology and Medicine* 27, no. 3 (1984): 361–366, doi:10.1353/pbm.1984.0033.

34. S. Finger and W. Zeitler, "Benjamin Franklin and His Glass Armonica: From Music as Therapeutic to Pathological," in Altenmüller, Finger, and Boller, *Music, Neurology, and Neuroscience: Historical Connections and Perspectives*.

35. "Explanation Sought for Teen Fainting Spells," *Stevens Point* (WI) *Daily Journal*, April 10, 1976, 11.

CONCLUSION

1. Y. Ikemi and S. Nakagawa "A Psychosomatic Study of Contagious Dermatitis," *Kyushu Journal of Medical Science* 13, no. 6 (1962): 335–350.

2. S. Roy, K. J. Petrie, G. Gamble, and M. A. Edwards, "Did a Nocebo Effect Contribute to the Rise in Special Education Enrollment Following the Flint, Michigan Water Crisis?," *Clinical Psychology in Europe* 5, no. 1 (2023).

3. G. A. Marlatt, B. Demming, and J. B. Reid, "Loss of Control Drinking in Alcoholics: An Experimental Analogue," *Journal of Abnormal Psychology* 81, no. 3 (1973): 233.

4. P. J. Jones, B. W. Bellet, and R. J. McNally, "Helping or Harming? The Effect of Trigger Warnings on Individuals with Trauma Histories," *Clinical Psychological Science* 8, no. 5 (2020): 905–917.

5. M. Sanson, D. Strange, and M. Garry, "Trigger Warnings Are Trivially Helpful at Reducing Negative Affect, Intrusive Thoughts, and Avoidance," *Clinical Psychological Science* 7, no. 4 (2019): 778–793, https://doi.org/10.1177/2167702619827018.

6. C. Blease, B. Colagiuri, and C. Locher, "Replication Crisis and Placebo Studies: Rebooting the Bioethical Debate," *Journal of Medical Ethics*, published online January 6, 2023, doi:10.1136/jme-2022-108672.

7. C. R. Blease, "Sharing Online Clinical Notes with Patients: Implications for Nocebo Effects and Health Equity," *Journal of Medical Ethics* 49, no. 1 (2023): 14–21, doi:10.1136/jme-2022-108413.

INDEX